Instant

Herbal Locator

by

Hanna Kroeger

Foreword

INSTANT HERBAL LOCATOR does not need a foreword. The author said, "I cannot keep all the herbals in my head." To facilitate the task of constant looking up for the most beneficial herb for a special purpose, Hanna has compiled this handy book for herself and for you.

Condition of Sale

This book is not made in juxtaposition of any product for the purpose of promoting that product.

The author is not guilty of any violation of this regulation made by the United States Food and Drug Administration.

The author makes no medical claim. The patient should consult a licensed physician for any condition that logically requires his/her services. This book is not intended as a substitute for proper medical care.

Americans

Americans are traditionally the "Do it Yourself" type. I saw a dentist painting his own living room over a holiday weekend; I noticed a lawyer fixing his own car engine; a farmer building a chapel for himself and his neighbors; I saw a woman building a greenhouse all by herself; a physician's wife raising chickens; a politician's wife raising the family's vegetables.

Americans are ingenious. Men can fix leaking roofs and dripping faucets. They can fix electrical wires and broken lamps. Women can bake and cook and in the same day be charming hostess. They are their own hairdressers, upholsterers, painters, and "fix-it-all's."

Why, then, are men and women so reluctant in helping themselves to radiant health with Herbs? The knowledge of the healing power in herbs is as old as men and women existed. Again I emphasize that herbs do not interfere with the work your physician does for you. Herbs work on your spiritual body, harmonizing, balancing, and uplifting.

I dedicate this book to my ingenious fellow man.
The Do-It-Yourself type. The American.

WHY DO
HERBS HEAL

The courtroom was small and yet it was not crowded. The main occupants were the twelve jury men and women. The benches to the right were for the defendant and the benches to the left were for the plaintiff.

The case was a trial against a successful and very spiritual man—a man of great integrity, a healer, chiropractor, a patriot, a minister, and most of all, the best herbalist I have ever found.

After lunch it was my turn to testify for the healer's works. For weeks I had prepared for possible questions, placing the questions in my scrapbook and finding answers which were short and precise so that not much time would be taken.

The first hour went by . . . I had passed the tricks and tricky questions of the D.A., along with his cunning remarks and humiliations, when out of the blue sky this gentleman asked, "And why do herbs heal?" I was completely unprepared for this question! These wonderful helpers of mankind heal, and I had never even questioned why.

A silence spread over the crowd and into this silence again the triumphant question was asked. "Rev. Kroeger, tell us why do herbs heal?" I needed time to ask our Lord and I needed silence to receive His answer. So, I asked the D.A., "If I tell you the truth, will you accept it?" He replied, "I will." I still needed more time and I said to him, "If you will accept the truth, then promise that you will not be angry with me." I then was given a chance of silence because his reply was delayed, and in this silence I heard our Lord speak· In a flash of a moment the tense atmosphere had broken. It was as if sunshine had spread over all of us. The D.A. broke the silence with his promise to accept the truth and not to be angry. "This is the truth," I was impressed to say. "Herbs heal the spiritual body. Herbs heal the aura; herbs heal the subtle vital energies of the physical body. Herbs do not interfere with your physicians' prescriptions but they go far beyond the healing of drugs by healing the spirit, by energizing the aura, by strengthening the Bio-Life power." Now I understood the Bible verse in which Christ said, "Do not tax rue and spikenard." Herbs belong to religion and not in a court room.

And the angelics had filled every corner of the room so much so that the tired judge lifted his head from the Life Magazine he was reading and partook in the conversation. From then I knew that the wholeness of our plants heal our spiritual bodies and reflect to our physical needs.

A

ABDOMEN (Distended without nausea)
Nutmeg
  ½ teaspoon in hot water.

ABDOMINAL TENDERNESS
Lindenflower Tea.

12 Herb Solution
  H-12—rub on navel.

ABSENSE OF ALL MORAL RESTRAINT
Anacardium (Cashew nut).

ACNE, ON FACE
Walnut Leaves

ACNE
Dandelion

Nettle

Strawberry Leaves
  Single or together as a tea

  Take 2 charcoal tablets before each meal daily.

  Avoid all chocolate.

ACHING BACK (lumbar region)
Poke Root

    ½ cup twice a day.

ACHING OF HEELS
Poke Root

    ½ cup twice a day.

ACID INDIGESTION
Yarrow Tea

    ½ cup twice a day.

ACHES, IN NECK (see stomach)
Magnesium

    in neck muscle

    in shoulder muscle

AGING
Sarsaparilla Root Dried

    The dried root of Sarsaparilla is alledged to prolong life and hinder premature aging. Bring one teaspoon of Sarsaparilla Root and a cup of cold water to a boil and then turn down and simmer for five minutes. Drink six ounces twice a day.

Thyme

Lavender

H-12

Sage is best

ALCOHOLISM
Thyme Tea helps to stop the desire.

AMOEBA
Jasmine Tea

    One Cup three times a day.

Ipecac (homeopathic)

Garlic
>	Three to six capsules daily.

Papaya Leaf
>	Eat one daily to protect and to help.

AMOEBIC DYSENTERY
Ipecac (homeopathic)

AMPUTATION, STUMP PAIN
Comfrey Root Tea

ANEMIA
Eggplant
>	It reduces enlarged spleen and increases red blood corpusles and hemoglobin. Eggplant is very good for anemia.

Pumpkin Seeds
>	Chew very well.

ANKLES, SWOLLEN
Potato Peelings
>	Simmer one handful peelings in two cups water for 15 minutes. Strain and take two tablespoons of this in a glass of water for fourteen days. After several days your legs and ankles should be at a more normal size. (3 times daily)

ANKLES, WEAK
Scotch Pine Tea Compresses
>	Make a strong tea and wrap around ankles.

ANTI-FAT
Bladderwrack in tablet form.

ANTI-SPASMATIC
Cinque Foil Tea
>	½ cup as needed.

Balm Leaf Tea
>	One cup as needed.

Caraway
> This is a very well known spice that mainly works on the stomach. It is anti-spasmatic, it improves appetite, subsides gastric distention, takes out phlegm and is generally useful for stomach disorders.

Scullcap

ANUS, BITING
Paeonia as a tea.

ANUS, BURNING
Iris-Blue Flag as a tea.

ANUS, ITCHING
Ground Ivy Tea
> 1 cup a day.

ANUS, PAINFUL
Ginger Tea
> ½ cup three times a day.

APATHY
Saw Palmetto (homeopathic)

APPETITE, LOSS OF:
Vitamin B-6

Vitamin B-12

APPETITE, LOSS OF
Calamus Root
> Chew a piece or boil in one quart of apple juice.

APPETITE FOR MEAT, LOSS OF:
Choline

APPETITE, LOSS OF (in children)
Cranberry Juice or sauce

Red Clover Tea

ARCHES, FALLEN
Comfrey Root Tincture
> Applied overnight on sole of feet

ARTERIES, HARDENING
Apple Tree Bark Tea

ARTHRITIC, DEFORMATION ON HANDS AND FEET
Warm Comfrey Root Compresses
> Heat a cabbage leaf and apply over night.

ARTHRITIS
Rumafix
> See special formulas.

ARTHRITIS
Oil of Wintergreen
> Rub on joints, also kerosene on joints. Eat Strawberries, cranberries and asparagus.

ASTHMA
Cranberry Juice Concentrate
> 1 teaspoon can stop an asthma attack. To make your own boil one pint water and one pound cranberries until done, then keep refrigerated. Dosage: one teaspoon.
>
> Grate Black Radish and add honey to it, take one teaspoon of this mixture before going to bed.
>
> Go on ½ day fast. The time you do not eat, drink 2 quarts of water. Soak fresh pineapples in two quarts of water for two hours. Drink from this fluid for the other half of the day; all you want. Do this for 10 to 14 days.
>
> Thyme Powder mixed with honey—take 1 teaspoon every hour.
>
> Wormwood
> Boiled in Applejuice.
>
> Gall bladder flush
>
> Elecampane and Quebracho

LEMON JUICE
2 tablespoons before each meal.

Sunflower Seeds
Take one quart of seeds, put in a half gallon of water and boil down to one quart of water. Strain, add one pint of honey and boil it down to a syrup. Give one teaspoon three times a day.

Wild Plum Tree Bark
Make syrup and take one tablespoon four times a day. Make a pillow and sleep with it. Good for hayfever too.

ASTHMA, ATTACK AFTER FIRST SLEEP
Spikenard Tea
1 teaspoon twice a day.

ASTHMA, IN CHILDREN
Thuja (homeopathic)

ASTHMA, THROUGH NERVOUSNESS
Dandelion Root and Leaves Tea

ASTHMA, WITHOUT ANXIETY
Ginger

Wild Plum Bark, Wild Cherry Bark
1 teaspoon to a cup of tea.

AURA CLEANSER
Rose petals

Cyani Flowers

Yarrow
Brew the above, steep, strain and add to bathwater.

B

BABY, HEALTHY
Squaw Vine

BACK, ACHING—LUMBAR REGION
Poke Root Tea
         2 cups a day—simmer root.

BACK ACHE
Affecting hips and sacrum (walks stooped)
         Horse Chestnut

BAD NATURED TUMORS—GENERAL
Prickly Pear

BAD NATURED TUMORS—ON LIPS
Juice of Milkweed
         Apply to lip.

BAD NATURED TUMORS—OF BREAST
Houseleek, Cottonwood Leaves
         Make Tea.

BACKWARD CHILDREN
Alfalfa Seed Tea

Dill added to food

BEDWETTING
Violet Leaf Tea

Bisort Tea

Equisetum as a tea.

BELCHING
Saw Palmetto Tea

BILEDUCT, SLUGGISH
Mugwort

Cheladonium
>½ cup before meals.

BILE, INCREASE
Garden Radish
>One before meals.

BLADDER INFECTION
Uva Ursi Tea

BLADDER INFECTION (bleeding and burning)
Marshmellow Root Tea

BLADDER PAIN
Marshmellow Root Tea

BLADDER SPASMS
Uva Ursi Tea
>One cup three times a day.

BLADDER STONES
Carrot Leaves
>Make tea.

BLADDER WEAK
Parsley Tea

Lathyrus—Chick Pea (homeopathic)

BLEEDING OF BOWELS
Cinnemon Tea.

BLEEDING, FEMALE
Yarrow and Plantain
>Equal parts, 3 cups of tea a day

Okra

BLEEDING
Shepards' Purse
> For intestinal bleeding, bleeding under the skin drink 1 cup twice a day.

Sesame Oil
> 2 teaspoons a day.

Yarrow Tea
> 1 cup a day.

BLEEDING, IN URINE
Comfrey Root

Dandelion Root

Marshmallow Root
> Mix and make a tea—2 teaspoons to a cup.

BLISTERS IN PALM
Ranunculus = Buttercup (homeopathic)

BLOATEDNESS
Fennel Tea.

Sage Tea

BLOATEDNESS
> 5 to 6 drops oil of Anise on 1 teaspoon of honey or water.

BLOOD CLEANSER
Mild: Sanicle—1 teaspoon to a cup of boiling water.

Mild: Red Clover—5 parts
        Chaparell—1 part

Harsh: Sassafras—1 teaspoon to a cup of boiling water

        Sheep Sorell—1 teaspoon to 1 cup of boiling water

        H-12

        Lemon juice, honey and water—6 oz. every 2 hours

BLOOD CLOTS
3 cups Red Clover Tea (very strong)

500 mg. of Vitamin C.

4 teaspoons wheatgerm oil (no butter or peanut oil)

also

> Take a piece of cotton cloth, sprinkle with salt and place over the site of the trouble.

BLOOD CIRCULATION
Rosemary and Chamomile Tea
> Hot before retiring.

Powdered Red Pepper
> In stockings.

BLOOD POISONING
Hyssop Tea
> 1 gallon a day for two days.

Bathe—boil 20 Peach leaves in 1 quart of boiling water for 10 minutes. Strain and put water in bath.

BLOOD PRESSURE—HIGH
Mistletoe and Angelica
> Two teaspoons each in 1 quart of boiling water. Drink 2 to 3 cups a day.

BLOOD PRESSURE
Garlic
> Equalizes blood pressure and makes elasticity of blood vessels. Take 3 to 6 capsules daily.

BLOOD PRESSURE—LOW
Cayenne Pepper

Apricots

Protein

> Add Cayenne pepper to your food, mix apricots and dark raisins and eat two tablespoons three times daily.

BLOOD PRESSURE STABILIZER
Shepards Purse Tea
>Two cups per day, one teaspoon of tea to a cup of boiling water.

BLOOD VESSELS, ENLARGED
Horse Chestnut Tea

BLOOD PURIFIER
Sassafras Tea

Burdock Tea

Red Clover Tea

Two tablespoons of Woodruff boiled in 1 quart grape juice. Drink 6 oz. twice daily for 3 weeks.

BLOOD PURIFIER FOR GLANDS
Hyssop
>(Bible "Wash me with Hyssop and make me White as snow.")

BLOOD PURIFIER FOR SKIN
Strawberry Leaves Tea

Primula Officinalis Tea

Nettle Tea

Ground Ivy Tea

mix them or each one by itself

BLOOD THINNER
Rosemary Tea

Red Clover (seeds and tops—make tea)

Sassafras

Burdock

Red Clover Tops
>Mix and drink 2 cups a day.
>1 teaspoon to a cup.

Primula Officinalis Tea

Nettle Tea

Dandelion Tea
> Mix and drink 2 cups a day.
> 2 teaspoons to a cup.

BLOOD URINE
Comfrey Root

Dandelion Root

Marshmallow Root
> Mix and make tea. 2 teaspoons to a cup.

BLOWING THE NOSE FREQUENTLY
Couch Grass Tea
> 1 tablespoon to a cup of water.
> Drink several cups a day.

BOILS
Calendula Oil (see oil recipe)
> Calendula Oil is for everything that needs healing.

BOILS AND PIMPLES
Nutmeg
> One third teaspoon of freshly ground nutmeg, one teaspoon honey and four or five ounces hot water. Drink this for three mornings in a row. Don't drink it for three days. Repeat this nine times.

Onion
> Put onion poultice over a boil to bring it to a head.

BONES, BROKEN
Take an orange towel and sleep on it, also do it
(When bones are healed and still give trouble.)

Wild Geranium as a tea.

Comfrey Root Tea

Bonemeal—three tablets three times a day.

BONES, TENDONS AND MUSCLE INJURIES
Comfrey Root Compresses

BONES, PAIN IN
Comfrey Root Tea

Comfrey Root Tincture

BONES, WEAK
Fenugreek Seed
> In tablet or capsule form

BOTULISM
Pokeroot—six parts

Sarsaparilla—three parts
> Make strong tea and give it by the tablespoon every ½ hour.

BOWELS, DROPPED
Prickly Ash Tea
> Two cups a day.

BRAIN CONGESTION
Cowslip Tea
> ½ cup several times a day.

BRAIN, SLUGGISH
Eyebright and/or

Gotu Kola

BREAST, LUMPS
Carrot Compresses

Ivory Soap
> Grate Ivory soap into warm, dissolved beeswax and apply overnight.

BREAST, PROBLEMS
Hard

Pokeroot
> Make strong tea compress over breast

Pain (in left breast)
Myrtle Tea
> Two cups a day.

Very Sensitive
Pokeroot Tea
> Drink two cups and also externally as a compress.

BREATHING DIFFICULTY
Black Tea
> A cup of black tea often removes breathing difficulty until you get
> a doctor's help.

BREATHING DIFFICULTY, CHORNIC
White Hellebore Tea

H-12

BRIGHTS DISEASE
Watermelon Seed Tea
> Make it strong and give two tablespoons every hour.

BRONCHIAL ASTHMA
Angelica Root Tea with honey

BRONCHIAL CONSTRICTION (cough)

BRONCHIAL INFECTION
Yerba Santa is a specific herb for it.

BRONCHIAL TROUBLE
Thyme Tea
> 1 tablespoon every hour

or

Fennel

Dandelion Leaves
> Mix equal parts and make a tea.
> Drink 3 to 4 cups a day.

BRONCHITIS
Daffodil

Lungwort

Plantain

   or

H-12

   also

Flaxseed Tea
> To a pint of tea add the juice of two lemons. Add three tablespoons of honey and take a teaspoon every half hour until relieved.

BRONCHITIS IN OLD AGE
White Hellebore

BRUISES
A handful of fresh crushed peach leaves applied as a poultice

Salomon Seal as a poultice

Daisy Tea and as a poultice

BURGER'S DISEASE
Nettle Root Compresses

Nettle Tea to drink

C

CALLUSES
Peppermint Oil—rubbed on.

CANCER, SKIN (Appalation Recipe)
Wood Sorrel Leaves
> Applied as a poultice is said to pull out the core of the cancer and hurts but heals.

Ground Ivy
> A low creeping plant used by the Irish to make a strong tea and drink it for skin cancer.

CANNOT BEAR . . .
Odors—Nux Vomica (homeopathic)

Light—Nux Vomica (homeopathic)

Noise—Nux Vomica (homeopathic)

CANNOT WALK ON UNEVEN GROUND
Tiger Lily

CATARACT
Cheddar Cheese

Vitamin B-2
> A Doctor in the East gives B-2 against cataract with excellent results.

Celandine

CATARRH
Cleaver Tea
> Several cups.

CATARRHAL DEAFNESS
Garlic

CELL BALANCER
Chaparell

CEREBRAL CONGESTION
Cowslip Tea
> 2 cups a day.

CHANGE OF LIFE
Black Cohosh—in capsules

Sarsaparilla—in capsules

Licorice Tea

Take the above as needed.

CHEST AFFLICTIONS
Nettle Tea

CHILDREN, BACKWARD
Alfalfa Seed Tea

Dill added to food

CHILDREN, DULL
Nettle Tea

H-12—5 drops a day.

CHILDREN'S FEVER
Gelsemium (homeopathic)

Echinacea (homeopathic)

CHOLERA
Tobacco

Zinc

CHOLESTEROL DEPOSITS
Alfalfa Sprouts

CIRCULATION, BLOOD
Rosemary and Chamomile Tea
        Hot before retiring.

Ground Red Pepper in socks

CIRCULATION TO PELVIC ORGANS
Tansy Tea
        ½ cup twice a day.

CIRCULATION, SLUGGISH
Comfrey Root Tea
        Soak one teaspoon in chopped root in 8 ounces of water overnight,
        then warm and drink it warm.

CIRCULATION TO UTERUS
Tansy Tea
> ½ cup twice a day.

CIRRHOSIS OF THE LIVER
Club Moss Compresses

CLAY COLORED STOOLS
Chickweed

Livah*

CLEARS COMPLEXTION
Barberries

Mountain Grape

COBALT 60
Mullein Leaves—2 cups a day.

COLD, HEAD
Myrtle
> Inhaling warm vapors relives pain caused by a severe cold. Preventative—Thyme Tea—1 cup a day, 1 teaspoon to a cup.

COLITIS
Comfrey Tea

Fenugreek Tea

COLLAPSE
White Hellebore

CONCENTRATION
Vitamin B-12, Folic Acid, Gotu Kola

CONGESTION, KIDNEY
Parsley Root Tea

CONSTIPATION
Flax Seed
>Soak overnight.

CONFUSION
Ginger Tea
>½ cup twice a day.

CONFUSED THOUGHTS
Club Moss

H-12

CONJUNCTIVITIS
Raw potato on eye.

CONSTIPATION DUE TO SLUGGISH LIVER
Barberry Tea
>1 cup with meals.

CO-ORDINATION, LACK OF
Ignatius Beans (homeopathic)

CORNS ON FEET, SENSITIVE
Ranunculus-Buttercup

CORNS
>Soak your feet in warm water for about 15 minutes then cut a small piece of lemon peel and place the inside of it against the corn, tying it on and let it stay there all night. Do this for several nights and the corn should lift out.

COUGH, DRY
>Cut onions, boil in vinegar for 15 minutes and add honey. Take 1 teaspoon every hour.

COUGH OF A CRAMPING NATURE
Thyme Tea

Primula Tea

Elder Tea

COUGH, OBSTINATE
Iceland Moss Tea

COUGH
Onion, red or yellow

Cherry Bark Tea

COUGH SYRUP
Mullein Leaves
> Mashed, boiled strained and add sugar cook down to a thick syrup.

COUGH, WHOOPING
Wild Cherry Bark—1 teaspoon

Sage—1 tablespoon
> In a pint of water and take 1 teaspoon 5 times daily

COURAGE
Vitamin C

Calcium

CRAMPS, LEGS
Club Moss Compress
> (place on feet) or in a pillow

> Calcium Lactate, B-1

CRAMPS IN SOLES AND PALMS
Ginger Tea

Curvature, Spine
Chlorine Herbs

H-12 Mixture applied to spine

D

DANDRUFF

Boil a handful of willow leaves, strain and wash your hair and scalp in it. Put a little of the tea aside and dampen the scalp every day a little. Found recipe in an old herb book. I was amazed over the results.

DEAFNESS, RHEUMATIC

Mistletoe (homeopathic)

DEBILITY

Ginger Tea—1 cup

DEBILITY OF LIMBS

Daisy Tea—2 cups a day.

Juniper branches

Boil for 45 minutes and add the fluid to bath water twice a week.

DEPRESSION

Black Snake Root

The Indians chewed this root to calm the nerves and to alleviate depression.

Daisy Tea

DIABETES

Dwarf Leaves—2 cups a day.

Devil's Claw in capsules

Blueberry Leaf Tea or

Blackberry Leaf Tea

Oat Straw Tea—boil and drink 4 cups a day

White Figs—make compresses over throat

SEE PHYSICIAN

DIARRHEA
Oak Bark Tea

Tea of Dried Blackberry Root or

Blackberry Juice

Slippery Elm

DIFFICULTY IN
Speaking and singing

  Sulfur

Taking a Deep Breath

  Iron

Digest Protein

  Sage Tea—one cup twice a day also Basil

Thinking

  Calcium

Diverticulitus
B-Complex from Rice Bran

DIURETIC
Parsley Root Tea

DIZZINESS
Mustard Seeds
    Chew 1 teaspoon of Mustard Seeds every morning.

DIZZY, HEAD FEELS DIZZY
Intoxication Yerba Santa Tea—one or two cups a day.

DUODENAL ULCER
Calamus Root
    Let sit in cold water overnight warm it in the morning, take 2 tablespoons six times a day.

    Comfrey Root Tea—2 cups a day.

DREAMS, TERRIFYING
Paeonis

DROPSY
Broom Tops—in capsules or as tea.
Potatoe Peelings—boil peelings and drink 6 ounces twice a day.
Elder Flowers—2 cups a day.
Horseradish in Apple Juice—½ cup 3 times a day.
> One half gallon Apple Cider plus a handful of parsley (crushed), a handful of Horseradish (crushed) and a tablespoon of Juniper Berries combined and let stand for 24 hours in a warm place. Drink a half glass three times a day before meals.

DRY MOTHER'S MILK
Cransbill Tea—(strong) massaged into breast

Sage Tea—3 cups a day

DRY MOUTH AND THROAT
Calamus Root—chew a small piece

DULL CHILDREN
Nettles

DUODENAL ULCER
Calamus Root Tea
> Root should stand in water overnight, warm it the next morning (Do Not Boil). Drink ½ cup four to five times daily.

H-12

DYSENTERY
Ipecac (homeopathic)

E

EARS, BURNING
Cayenne Pepper

EAR, GENERAL
Violet Root

EAR ACHE
Pepper
> Moisten cloth with oil, sprinkle with black pepper and apply outside of ear like a compress.

EAR, GLAND SWOLLEN
Flax Seed (Ground)
> Mix Flax Seed with salt, put between layers of cloth and apply.

EAR, INNER
Horsetail
> One handful, boil and strain. Add to your bath. Soak for 20 minutes.

EAR, PAIN
Plantain
> Going from one ear through the head to the other ear.

EAR, RINGING IN
Iris-Blue Flag (homeopathic)

EAR, SHOOTING PAIN IN
Violet Leaf Tea

EAR, STINGING
Violet Leaf Tea

EAR SWELLING (behind)
Pepper
> Moisten cloth, sprinkle with black pepper and apply.

ECZEMA
Strawberry Leaf Tea

ECZEMA, BEHIND THE EAR
Club Moss

ECZEMA IN CHILDHOOD
Pansy Tea (Viola Triealas)

ECZEMA, ERUPTIONS AND BLISTERS
OVER JOINTS AND FINGERS
Evening Primrose Oil

ECZEMA, SCALP
Pansy Tea (Viola Triealas)

EMOTION
Ignatius Bean (homeopathic)

EMOTIONAL SENSITIVITY
Thuja Tea or homeopathic form

EMOTIONAL UPSET
Meadow Sweet Tea
        1 cup sweetened with honey.

ENERGY
Vitamin B-1, B-Complex, Lecithin, Pantothenic Acid

ENLARGED BLOOD VESSELS
Horse Chestnut Tea

ENLARGED GLANDS
Poke Root
        ½ cup twice a day.

ENLARGED UTERUS
Yarrow Tea

ENVIRONMENTAL POISON
Willow Leaf Tea—2 cups or more.

EPILEPSY
Mistle (homeopathic)

Valerian Root

ESOPHAGUS, TUMEROUS
Cheese Button Weed
    Drink 3 cups a day in small sips.

ESOPHAGUS, ULCERATED
Cheese Button Weed Tea

Calamus Root—Chew a piece.

EUSTACHIAN TUBE
Black Pepper from outside (see Ears)

EUSTACHIAN TUBE, CATARRH
Rose Petal Tea—2 cups a day.

EUSTACHIAN TUBE, STUFFED
Alfalfa Seed Tea—several cups.

EXHAUSTION, NERVOUS
Silicon Herbs (see back of book)

EYE, ACHING
Calcium Fluoride

Athrophy of the Optic Nerve
    Tobacco Water—Bathe in.

Burning
    Eyebright Tea—2 cups a day.
    Vitamins A and B-2.

Conjunctivitis
    Raw Potatoe on eye

Dirty Yellow Color
  Celandine (homeopathic)

Eyelids, Heavy
  Violet Leaf Tea

Farsighted
  Protein—lack of, you need more.

Fibrilation
  Viatmin B-1.

Hemorrhage
  Linden Flower Tea—
        Drink cool, two cups a day.

Inflamed
  Red Potato Slices—applied to eye.
  White Lily Leaves—applied to eye.
  Castor Oil—apply to eye.
  Elder Flower Tea—apply externally and drink internally.
  Eyebright Tea

Loss of Eyesight from Diabetes
  Zinc
  Paprika (Hungarian is best)

Loss of Eyesight from Tobacco
  Vitamin B-12
  Folic Acid

Muscular Weakness
  Linden Flower Tea
        Drink two cups a day, cool.

Pressured
  Poke Root Tea
        One cup twice a day.
  Red Clover Tea
  Manganese

Eye, Retina Bleeding
  Vitamin C
  Bioflavenoids
  Rutin
  Vitamin B-1
  Raw Potato Compresses
  Paprika (Hungarian is best)
      One teaspoon on your food three times a day.

Sensation of Gauze before the Eyes
  Linden Flower Tea—Two cups a day.

Strengthener
  Angelica Root Tea—½ cup twice a day.
  Maple Syrup

Stye
  Eyebright—If possible in homeopathic form.

Tired
  Vitamins A, B-2, C, and E with ½ to 1 teaspoon of Pure Maple Syrup.
  Eyebright for trace minerals.

Trauma (hard blow)
  Comfrey Root Compresses

Twitching Eyelid
  Elder Flower Tea
  Vitamin B-6

Weak
  Rue Tea—two cups a day.

FACIAL NEURALGIA
Raw Plantain Juice—over painful area.

FAINTING
Lavender Tea

Vitamin E, B-Complex, B-6

Manganese

FAINT—ALL GONE FEELING
Blood Root Tea—one cup twice a day.

FALLOUT
Cinnamon on burnt toast

Cloves with Vitamin C

Willows Leaf Tea—2 cups a day

FAT, ANTI-FAT
Bladderwrack in tablet form

FEAR OF EXAMINATION
Anacardium (cashew nuts)—chew nuts.

FEAR
Rosemary Tea
Cinnamon Tea
Lavender Tea
        Equal parts for Tea

FEELING OF INTOXICATION
Valerian Root Tea

FEELING TOO COLD
Seaweed or Kelp and Cayenne in hot water

FEELING TOO HOT
Motherwort as a Tea.

FEELING AS IF SOUL AND BODY ARE SEPARATE
Thuja (homeopathic)

FEMALE TROUBLE, INFECTION
Nettle Tea
>Known for it's anti-fungal and anti-viral Properties.

FEVER (GENERAL)
Melissa Tea—2 cups

Feverfew Tea—2 cups

Garlic—in capsules

Herbal Spice Tea
>Use equal parts: Cardamon, Cloves and a little Black Pepper.

FEVER WITH FLU
Onion
>Make onion soup, this soup will bring Vitamin C to work.

FEVER IN CHILDREN
Yellow Jasmine

Gelsemium (homeopathic)

Echinacea (homeopathic)

FEVER, INTERMITTENT
Holly Tea

FEVER, REDUCED
Pleurisy Root

FEVER, TIC
Chaparell
>Three tablets three times a day for one month.

FIBROID TUMOR
Golden Rod as a Tea

also drink:
>Calundula—2 parts
>Yarrow—1 part
>Nettle—1 part
>Mix and use 1 quart a day for 4 weeks

FINGERS, SWOLLEN
Iodine Herbs (see back of book)

FINGERNAILS, FLATTENED
Iron Deficiency

Thin
  Sulphur Deficiency

Split
  Mineral Deficiency

FINGERTIPS CHAPPED
Ranunculus—Buttercup (homeopathic)

FORGETFULNESS
Rosemary Tea

Eyebright in capsules or tablets.

Sage on a slice of buttered rye bread.

FRIGHTENED (VERY EASILY)
Elder Flowers
        One small cup twice a day.

FROSTBITE
Calamus Root
        Soak in Calamus Root Tea.

FUNGUS
Asparagus
        2 tablespoons twice a day.

Concord Grape Juice
        3 glasses a day.

G

GALL BLADDER
Chronic Trouble
  Chelidonium (homeopathic)

Obstruction
  Chelidonium (homeopathic)

Pain
  Chelidonium (homeopathic)

GANGRENE
Enchinacea in capsules

Willow Leaves applied directly as compress.

Tobacco Tea as compress (American Indian).

GAS PAIN
Rue Tea (Not During Pregnancy)
        One cup with meals.

GASTRIC INDIGESTION
Copper Herbs (see back of book)

GASTRO-DUODENAL CATARRAH
Blood Root Tea
        ½ cup twice a day.

GLAND BALANCER
Mallow Leaf Tea
        2 cups a day.

GLANDS, ENLARGED
Poke Root Tea
        ½ cup twice a day.

GLAND FOOD
Yams

Sweet Potatoes

Sesame Seeds

Sunflower Seeds

Avacado without oil or butter

GLAND PURIFIER FOR THE BLOOD
Hyssop Tea
(Bible "Wash me with Hyssop and make me white as snow.")

GLAND STIMULANT
Barberries
In capsules or as a tea.

GLANDS, SWOLLEN
Plantain Leaves
Boil and mix with salt, then use as a compress.

Majorum

Plantain
Make an oil with these and apply. Plantain neutralizes poisons.

GLANDULARS IN HERBOLOGY
Dandelion Root
Stimulates glands.

Alfalfa Seed Tea
Nourishes glands.

Yucca
Similar to cortisone—adrenal gland food.

GLANDULAR SYSTEM (Good for)
Mullein Leaf Tea—2 cups a day.

GLANDULAR Tissue (strengthener)
Saw Palmetto (homeopathic) or in capsules

GLANDULAR WEAKNESS
Sage Tea—1 cup daily.

GLUTEAL MUSCLE EMACIATED
Lathyrus (homeopathic)

Chick Pea (homeopathic)

GLAUCOMA
Yellow Onion
> Place a thin slice over closed eyes until tears come. Remove and wash eyes in fresh water.

GOITER
Poke Root Tea—2 cups a day.

GONORRHEA
Black Walnut Tea—4 cups a day.

GOUT
Hydrangia Root Tea—2 cups a day.

Comfrey Root Tea—3 times a day.

GREYING OF HAIR
Sage Tea

Nettle Tea
> Rinse through hair.

GRIPPING IN INTESTINES
Coriander
> Chew five seeds or brew as a tea.

GUM DISEASE
Verbena
> Make a strong tea and hold a small portion in mouth several times a day.

Parsley Tea
>Use as Verbena.

GUMS, SORE
>Hold Hyssop Tea in mouth several times a day.

H

HAIR BRITTLE
Nettle Tea
>Wash hair with it.

HAIR COLOR (to retain the natural color)
Iodine Herbs (see back of book)

HAIR, COLORING
Nettle Root

HAIR, FALLING OUT DIET
>Could be signs of an underactive thyroid.
>Eat high protein, no sugar at all and plenty of yogurt.

HAIR, GREY
Sage Tea

Nettle Tea
>Rinse hair with.

HAIR LOSS
Nettle Tea—drink.

Sarsaparilla

Wormwood Tea
>Drink and rinse with cooled tea. Brew two tablespoons in one quart
>of water for 25 minutes, cool before moistening the scalp.

Silicon Herbs (see back of book)

HAIR TONIC
Nettle Tea

HAIR VERY GREASY
Wild Hops

Vitamin B-2

WHITE SCALY DANDRUFF
Nettle

Willow Leaf Tea

HAIR LOSS PREVENTIVE
Rosemary
> One pint of boiling water over one ounce of Rosemary and mix into solution of two tablespoons baking soda, strain and use as a hair rinse to prevent premature baldness.

> Boil a spoonful of Southernwood in a pint of water for three minutes.

HALLUCINATIONS
Anacardium (Cashew Nut)
> Chew nuts thoroughly.

HALLUCINATIONS AT NIGHT
Valerian Root Tea
> One or two cups at bedtime.

HARDENING OF THE ARTERIES
Apple Tree Bark

HARD OF HEARING
Bethroot Tea—2 cups daily.

HAY FEVER
Clover Tea

Red Onion Soup

Spikenard Tea

Wild Plum Tree Bark
> Two ounces to one quart of water, boil down to one cup and add one cup of honey or maple or brown sugar and boil down again. Take one tablespoon four times a day or as needed.

Cherry Bark Tea—2 cups daily.

HAYFEVER WITH ASTHMA
Damask Rose
> Two tablespoons four times daily.

HAYFEVER WITH PROFUSE YELLOW DISCHARGE
Fenugreek

Nettle Tea

HEADACHE (radiating from one point)
Black Tea—one cup.

HEADACHE (with nausea)
Iris-Blue Flag (homeopathic)

HEADACHE
Lady's Slipper Tea
(also called Nerve Root)

Lavender Tea

Lavender Oil
> To temples. NOT TO BE TAKEN INTERNALLY.

Lavender
> Applied hot will relieve almost any local pain.

Guarana Tea
> One cup when headache starts.

Back of Head
  liver and gallbladder

Front of Head
  Kidney, bladder

Middle
Intestinal

On One Side or The Other Side
Allergic reaction to something

Right Sided
Celadine Tea—1 cup a day.

HEAD COLD
Myrtle

Inhaling warm vapors relieves pain caused by severe cold.
Apply to forehead as a compress.

HEAD FEELS DIZZY, INTOXICATION
Yerba Santa Tea—1 or 2 cups.

HEALTHY BABIES
Squaw Vine

HEALTHY MOTHERS
Squaw Vine

Raspberry Leaf Tea—2 cups daily.

HEARING SHRILL, HIGH PITCHED SOUNDS
Violet Leaf Tea—2 cups a day.

HEARING DIFFICULTY (Rheumatic)
Garlic Oil

Drench some cotton with garlic oil and put into ear.
Wood Bethany—2 cups a day.

HEARING LOSS
Beth Root Tea—2 cups a day.

HEARING, RHEUMATIC DEAFNESS
Mistletoe (homeopathic)

HEARING, RINGING IN EAR
Iris-Blue Flag (homeopathic)

HEART, BROKEN
Balm Gilead Buds
        Carried in pocket or as a tea.

HEART BURN
Slippery Elm Tea

HEART ENLARGED
Asparagus
        Two tablespoons twice a day. Also B_1

HEART FOOD
Heartwarmer*

HEART, FIBRILATION
Cinnamon Sticks—Chew.

Rosemary Tea

Lemon Juice with Cloves

Put face in coal water.

HEART, IRREGULARITY
Basil Tea—or in capsules.

HEART MUSCLE
Hawthorne Berry Tea
        Two or three cups daily.

Rosemary Tea—2 cups a day.

HEART, NERVOUS
Rue Tea (Not During Pregnancy)

HEART, PALPITATIONS
Cloves in lemon juice
> Boil cloves in fresh or frozen lemon juice.
> Take one teaspoon in four ounces of water several times a day.

HEART STRENGTHENER
Cowslip—2 parts
Lavender—1 part
> Make tea using 1 teaspoon per cup and drink two to three cups a day.

HEART VALVES
Blue Malva Flower Tea
> One cup twice a day for six weeks.

HEAVINESS IN STOMACH
Ginger Tea

Violet Leaf Tea

HEAVINESS OF EYELIDS
Violet Leaf Tea

HEELS, ACHING
Poke Root

HEMORRHAGE FROM BLADDER
Peach Tree Bark Tea—3 cups a day.

Comfrey Root Tea—3 cups a day.

HEMORRAHAGE, FEMALE
Plantain
Yarrow
> Equal parts mixed and make a tea—3 cups a day.

HEMORROIDS, GENERAL
Vitamin B-6, Calcium, Chlorophyll, Smart Weed

Painful and Hot
  Ginger Tea

General
  Collinsonia Tea or in capsules.

  Dandelion Root Tea
    Brewed 15 minutes and drink two cups daily.

  Garlic
    Oil a clove and insert it into the rectum each night for several nights
    in a row.

  Cranberries
    Make a poultice over external hemorrhoid.

  Almonds
    Eat three a day to prevent and eliminate hemorrhoids.

  Potatoe
    Slice and dip in oil to lubricate and insert it into rectum

HEPATITIS, INFECTIOUS
Calendula (Marigold) Tea
    Calendula Tea and fresh Juice with distilled water and honey to
    taste. Drink one quart or more a day for a week. No fried foods,
    alcohol and keep warm.

HERNIA
Mistletoe
Horsetail
    Combine and apply as poultice over night.

HEROIN DEPOSITS
Chaparell Tea—Two cups a day or in capsules.

Tobacco Leaf Tea
    Add to bath water.

HERPES, GENERAL
Buckbean Tea—1 cup a day.

Club Moss

Ranunculus (homeopathic)

HERPES ZOSTER
Houseleek
> In soup or salad.

Iris Blue Flag (homeopathic)

B-Complex, B-1, Magnesium, Calcium

HERPES II
Blister type
> Ranunculus (homeopathic)
> Black Walnut Tea

HERPES LABIALIS
(with itching and sensation of heat)
Nettle Tea

HIGH BLOOD PRESSURE (due to Kidney)
Club Moss Tea

HOARSENESS
Ginger Tea with honey

Plantain Tea
> (Strong) sip it, it neutralizes poison.

HOME SICKNESS
Cayenne Pepper
> Added to food or sprinkle in shoes.

HOOKWORM
Homeopathic Remedy

also

> Two cups strong Thyme Tea will Paralyze Hookworms
> ½ hour later a good dose of Epsom salt

HORMONE, FEMALE
Black Cohosh

Rice Polishing

HORMONE, MALE
Sarsaparilla

Brewers Yeast

HORMONE SUPPLY
Pumpkin Seeds

HUMMING AND ROARING IN EARS
Club Moss Tea

HUNGER WITH NAUSEA
Valerian Root Tea—as needed.

HYPERACTIVE CHILDREN
Thyme Tea
> Two cups a day, one teaspoon to a cup.

HYSTERIA
Motherwort Tea
> One cup twice a day if connected with female trouble.

Passion Flowers—1 cup twice a day.

Sodium

Wood Bethony

HYSTERIA, CONNECTED WITH FEMALE TROUBLE
Motherwort Tea
> One cup twice a day.

HYSTERICAL FLATULANCE
Valerian Root Tea—or in capsules.

HYSTERICAL SPASMS IN STOMACH
Valerian Root Tea—or in capsules.

H-12—Rub in stomach.

HYDROCEPHALUS
Helleborus Tea
> One teaspoon four times a day.

I

ILL AFFECTS OF VACCINATION
Thuja (homeopathic)

ILL NATURED TUMORS
Blood Cleanser*

12 Root Formula—H-12

ILL NATURED TUMOR IN THE FEMALE ORGANS
Calendula

Yarrow

Nettle

ILL NATURED TUMOR IN KIDNEYS
Cheladonium

Golden Rod

Nettle

ILL NATURED TUMOR IN LIVER
Calamus Root
        ½ cup twice daily.
Golden Rod, Golden Seal, Cloves

ILL NATURED TUMOR IN LUNG
Garlic

Rose Hips

Rosemary

Echinacea

Thyme

ILL NATURED TUMOR IN PANCREAS
Calamus Root
> ½ cup four times a day.

H-12 Compresses

ILL NATURED TUMORS ON THE TONGUE
H-12 Compresses

Cheladonium

Cheese Button Weed

ILL NATURED TUMOR IN STOMACH
H-12 Compresses

Calendula

Nettle Tea

ILL NATURED TUMOR ON VOICE BOX
Cheese Button Weed

IMPETIGO
(especially over face and scalp)
Pansy Tea
> And/or as a rinse.

IMPOTENCE
Fenugreek Seed Tablets

INCREASE BILE
Garden Radish
> One before meals.

INDIFFERENT TO LIFE
Poke Root Tea—1 cup a day.

INDIGESTION
Summer Savory—add to food.

Anise Seed

Fennel Seed

Corriander
> Mix Equal parts together and make tea.

Yarrow Tea
> One cup twice a day.

INDESTION (chronic)
Slippery Elm Tea

INFANT COLIC
Caraway Seed Tea

INFECTED SKIN
White Pond Lily—apply to skin.

INFECTION
Parsley

Black Radish

INFECTION, FEMALE TROUBLE
Nettle Tea
> It is known that Nettle has anti-fungal, anti-viral properties.

INFECTION, VIRUS
Calendula Tea

INFECTIOUS HEPATITIS
Calendula (marigold) Tea and fresh lemon juice with distilled water and honey to taste. Drink one quart or more a day of the fresh lime juice for a week. Keep warm and eat no fried foods or alcoholic beverages.

INFLAMED NERVES (Very painful)
Peppermint Tea

Peppermint lotion

INFLAMATION OF EYE AND EYELID
Elder Flower Tca
>Externally also.

INJURIES TO TENDONS, BONES AND MUSCLES
Compresses of Comfrey

INJURIES TO DEEPER TISSUES
Daisy Tea—2 to 3 cups a day.

INJURIES TO NERVES
Daisy Tea—2 to 3 cups a day.

INJURIES TO SINEW, TENDONS AND JOINTS
Comfrey Root Compresses
Arnica is best.

INNER EAR
Horsetail
>One handful, boil and strain, then add to your bath. Soak for 20 minutes.

INSECT BITES
Sage Tea—rub it on.

INSOMNIA
Squaw Vine Tea

Raspberry Tea

INSOMNIA DUE TO WORRY
Prickly Ash Leaf Tea
>One cup at bedtime.

INSOMNIA IN INFANT
Passion Flower Tea
>One teaspoon of tea to a cup of water.

INSOMNIA IN AN AGED
Passion Flower Tea
>One cup at bedtime.

INSUFFICIENT THYMUS SECRETION
Copper Herbs—(see back of book)

INTERMITTENT FEVER
Holly Tea

INTESTINAL Catarrh
Ginger Tea

INTESTINE, GRIPPING IN
Coriander
>Chew 5 seeds or brew tea.

INTESTINAL MUCOUS
Garlic in capsules.

INTOXICATION, FEELING OF
Valerian Root Tea

ITCHING, INTENSE
Ranunculus—Buttercup (homeopathic)

ITCHING, INTOLERABLE
Pansy Tea
>One to three cups per day.

J

JAUNDICE
Golden Seal

Golden Rod

Cloves

  and

Fresh Lime Juice in Distilled Water

JAUNDICE IN CHILDREN
Hops Tea

Chamomile Tea

JERKING, CONSTANT
Valerian Root - in capsules.

Vitamin B-6

JOINT, TENDON AND SINEW, INJURIES TO
Comfrey Root Compresses

JOINTS, STIFF AND SWOLLEN
Burdock Root
  Boil it in milk and make a compress.

JOINTS, SWOLLEN
Wrap in grated cabbage overnight.

JOINTS FEEL WEAK
Ginger Tea
  Pinch of grated ginger in one cup boiling water sweetened with honey.

K

KIDNEY, BLEEDING
Watermelon Seed Tea

Magnesium

KIDNEY, CATARRHAL (Inflamation)
Juniper Berries

KIDNEY, CONGESTION
Verbena Tree

Parsley Root Tea

KIDNEY FUNCTION IMPAIRED
Magnesium

KIDNEY GRAVEL
Verbena Tea

Broom Top Tea

KIDNEY STONES
Chamomile and Knotgrass

KIDNEY STONES
1 tablespoon Dandelion Root (dried)

1 quart Apple Juice
        Boil for 10 minutes, strain and drink six ounces three times a day.

KIDNEY TROUBLE
Cornsilk Tea—3 cups a day.

KIDNEY TROUBLE (chronic)
Couchgrass Tea—3 cups a day.

KNEES KNOCK AGAINST EACH OTHER
Lathyrus—Chick Pea (homeopathic)

KNEES, SWOLLEN
Raw Poultice
> Grate two cups of cabbage, very fine—wrap in cloth and apply overnight for several nights in a row.

L

LACTATION
Lentils
> Eat them.

LACTATION, INCREASE IN MILK
Blessed Thistle Tea

LACTATION, INCREASE IN QUALITY
Alfalfa Tea

LACK OF MAGNETIC-ELECTRICAL ENERGIES
Iodine Herbs—(see back of book)

LACK OF PEPSIN
Hops Tea
> Before meals.

LACK OF SULPHUR
Fennel Seed
> Chew or make tea.

LARYNGITIS
Arnica Tincture
> Three to four drops in 1 tablespoon warm water several times a day.

> Violet Leaf Tea
> Drink or gargle.

Laryngitis, (chronic)
Thuja (homeopathic)

LARYNX, TICKLING
Red Onions

LEAD POISONING
Ground Ivy Tea—2 cups a day.

LEGS, BLUE IF HANGING DOWN
Lathyrus - Chick Pea (homeopathic)

LEG CRAMPS
Club Moss
> As a compress or in a pillow.

Lycopdium

Cramp Bark Tea

Club Moss
> Wrap around leg as a compress.

LEG TROUBLE
Male Fern
> Foot baths.

LEG TROUBLE, PARALYTIC WITH PAINS
Scullcap.

LEG TROUBLE, PAIN AT NIGHT
Could be lead poisoning or Cadmium Poison.

LEGS, SWOLLEN
Lady's Mantle.

LEUKEMIA
Okra

Sulphur Herbs (see back of book)

CANNOT BEAR, LIGHT
Nux Vomica (homeopathic)

LIMBS, PARALYTIC WITH PAINS
Scullcap Tea
>Or in capsule form. Drink several cups a day.

LIVER, CIRRHOSIS
Club Moss
>Compresses to the liver.

LIVER, CLEANSER
Chaparell Tea or in capsules.

LIVER, CONGESTION
Verbena Tea
>Two cups per day.

LIVER, CONSTIPATION DUE TO
Barberry Tea
>One cup with meals.

LIVER, CUTTING PAIN
Iris-Blue Flag (homeopathic is best)

LIVER, DAMAGE
Dandelion Leaves and stems of but not the flowers.

LIVER ENLARGED
Dandelion Tea
>Or fresh in salads.

LIVER ENLARGED AND TENDER WITH LOTS OF WIND
Senna

Chamomile

LIVER FOOD
Dandelion Leaves

Chelidonum (homeopathic)

LIVER, HARDENING OF
Golden Rod

Golden Seal

Cloves

Tradename—Livah*

LIVER PAIN
Yams

Yucca Tablets
> Pain in right side.

LIVER STRENGTHENER
Dandelion Root Tea

LIVER, SWOLLEN
Golden Rod

Golden Seal

Cloves

Tradename—Livah*

Fresh squeezed Lime Juice (2)
Distilled Water, 1 quart
Honey to taste
Drink a quart or more a day for seven days. Do not chill! Drink at room temperature. Do not eat *any* fried foods or alcoholic beverages and do keep your feet warm.

LOSS OF. . .
Alkali Reserves
  Vitamin B-1

Apple Cider Vinegar
    Two teaspoons in one cup of water with honey.

    Appetite
        Vitamins B-6, B-12

    Appetite for Meat Dishes
        Choline

    Breath Under Slightest Exertion
        See Physician
        Vitamin B-1

    Concentration
    Vitamin B-12, Folic Acid

    Courage
        Vitamin C, Calcium

    Energy
        Vitamin B-1, B-Complex, Lecithin, Pantothenic Acid

    Eyesight from Tobacco
        Vitamin B-12, Folic Acid

    Eyesight From Diabetes
        Zinc and Paprika (Hungarian is best)

    Hair
    Silicon Herbs (see back of book)

    Self-Confidence
        Club Moss

    Temperature
        Vitamin B-Complex, Kelp for Trace Minerals

    Willpower
    Calcium

LOW BLOOD SUGAR
Iron Herbs (see back of book)

Oil of Sassafras
>Rub in three drops Oil of Sassafras on the sole of each foot twice a day for four weeks.

>Ferrous Phosphate—Cell Salt #4

LOW OPINION OF YOURSELF
H-12 (see back of book)

LOW VITALITY
H-12 (see back of book)

LSD OVERDOSE/RESIDUE
Chaparell in tablet form

LUMP IN OVARIES
Calendula—2 parts
Plantain—1 part
Yarrow—1 part
>Make and drink tea. 1 quart a day for 4 weeks.

LUMP IN THROAT (Globus Hystericus)
St. Ignatius Bean (homeopathic)

LUMP IN THROAT
Blue Malva
>Let sit overnight in cold water.

LUNG CONGESTION
Water
>Aerate pure water by beating it with an eggbeater, drink it at once.

LUNG, COUGH
Lungwort Tea
>One to four cups a day.

LUNG, PHLEGM
Lungwort Tea
>One to four cups a day.

LUNG STRENGTHENER
Calamus Root

Yarrow

LUNG, WEAK
Lungwort Tea
>One to four cups a day.

LUPUS
Thuja (homeopathic)

Lymph Cleanser

Hyssop tea
>Two quarts a day or more for three days.

LYMPH GLANDS, DISEASED
Echinacea
>Two capsules twice a day.

LYMPH GLANDS ENLARGED
Poke Root Tea

LYMPH GLANDS, SWOLLEN
Lettuce

Basil

LYMPHATIC TROUBLE
Burdock Root Tea
>Two cups a day.

M

MAGNETISM, INCREASES IT
Mistletoe (homeopathic)

MALICIOUS
Anacardium (homeopathic)

MANIA
Horsetail (Cashew Nut)

MARROW OF BONES, STRENGTHEN
Yarrow Tea

MEASLES, FIRST STAGE
Eyebright

MEASLES, LATER ON
Pulsatilla

Alfalfa Seeds

Linden Blossoms

MEDITATION, AID FOR DEEPER
Lavender Tea

MELANCHOLY
Basil

> Keep in open bowl in the room to dispel Melancholy for the aroma tends to make people happy. Also season food with it.

> Club Moss (homeopathic)

> Vanilla Bean
> Cut one Vanilla Bean into pieces and boil in one pint of water. Drink six ounces two or three times a day.

MEMORY
Rosemary Tea

Eyebright Tablets

Sage on a slice of buttered Rye bread.

MENNINGITIS

Take a couple of Aloe Vera Leaves about six inches long, wash and cut in small pieces. Add three times the amount of water and simmer for ten minutes. Add two tablespoons honey or more to taste and simmer for another five minutes. Cool, strain and give one tablespoon to adult every hour and to a child one teaspoon every hour. The sicker you are the smaller the dosage.

Golden Seal
Scullcap
> Make tea to use for enemas.

MENOPAUSE

Yarrow—in capsules.

Black Cohoch—in capsules.

Rue Tea—2 cups a day.

Calcium Magnesium

Vitamin D
> Needed in adequate amounts or a deficiency causes nervousness, irritability, headaches, depression and arthritic problems may develop.

A high potency B-Complex taken one to three times a day further supports the nervous system and a daily intake of Vitamin E has been known to eliminate hot flashes and night sweats.

MENSIS, REGULATOR

Pulsatilla (homeopathic)

MENSTRUAL CRAMPS, RELIEVED

Motherwort

Crampbark
> One cup tea as needed.

MENSTRUAL DIFFICULTIES

Blue Cohosh—2 capsules needed.

MENSTRUAL FLOW, PROMOTES

Motherwort Tea

MENSTRUAL FLOW, SCANTY

Thyme Tea

MENSTRUAL TROUBLE, NO FLOW

Yarrow Tea—2 cups a day.

MENSTRUATION WITH CLOTS

Shepard's Purse
Two cups a day, one teaspoon to a cup of boiling water.

MENSTRUATION TOO FREQUENT AND COPIOUS

Shepard's Purse—2 cups a day.

MENSTRUATION, DISTURBED BECAUSE OF EMOTIONS

Tiger Lily (homeopathic)

MENTAL ALERTNESS

Bee Pollen
One Teaspoon a day.

MENTAL BOUYANCY

Alfalfa Seed Tea or in tablet form.

MENTAL EXHAUSTION

Sage

Lecthin

MENTAL DEPRESSION
Cleaver Tea

MENTAL DULLNESS
Hawthorne
>   In tablets or as a tea.

Eyebright
Dulse
>   Equal parts and make tea.

MENTAL HEALTH
Iodine Herbs (see back of book)

MENTAL INSTABILITY
Agar
Sorrel
>   Make tea and drink.

MENTAL STRENGTH
Iodine Herbs (see back of book)

MENTAL UPSET
Meadowsweet Tea
>   Two cups a day.

METALIC POISON
Pumpkin Seed

Okra

Rhubarb Root

Cayenne Pepper

Dulse

Peppermint

Metaline* Tradename

Vitamin C

Squash

Mexican Raw Sugar
>   One teaspoon several times a day until symptoms subside.

Strawberries

Green Beans

Zucchini
>Eat exclusively for three days to get rid of metalic poison.

MIGRAINE
Vervain Tea

Gurana—at the start of a headache.

Lavender Oil on Forehead.

MONONUCLEOSIS
Red Raspberry Leaf Tea

Leaf Lettuce Water/Tea

MOODINESS
Mallow Leaves as a tea.

MORNING SICKNESS
Peach Leaf Tea

MORPHINE HABIT
Oats

Celery Root called *celeriac*.

MOTHERS MILK (to dry up)
Cranesbill
>Strong tea over breast.

Sage Tea
>Three cups a day.

MOUTH BLISTERS
Sage
Arnica Violet
>Make tea, hold in mouth and drink.

MOUTH BURNING
Poppy Seed Tea
>Drink and hold in mouth several times a day.

MOUTH, DRY
Calamus Root
>Chew a small piece.

MOUTH ODOR
Chew Juniper Berries

Gargle with Rosemary Tea.

MOUTH ULCERS
Sage or
Willow Leaves
>Chew.

Blackberry Leaf Tea
>Hold in mouth.

MUCOUS
Oranges
>The mucous cleansers of the stomach, ears, head and sinuses if taken in the following manner: One glass of fresh squeezed orange juice followed by the same amount of distilled water. DO NOT MIX. First drink the orange juice, then follow with the water. Do this as often as you want, ten times a day or so. NO OTHER FOODS should be taken for two days. Do this two days in a row three times a year.

MUCOUS SOLVENT
Fenugreek

Southernwood

In Bronchi, Rattling
  Garlic

In Lungs
  Calamus Root Tea

MULTIPLE SCLEROSIS
Thyme Tea

MUMPS
Poke Root Tea
>   One cup three times a day.

Linden Flower Bath
>   Handful of Flowers, brew, strain and add to bath.

MUMPS AFTER SECOND STAGE
Pulsatilla (homeopathic)

Gotu Kola

Linden Blossom Tea

MUMPS RESIDUE
Gotu Kola in capsules.

MUSCLES
Aches in Shoulder
  Magnesium

Cramps
  Vitamin B-1, B-2, E, Caccium Lactate

Calves Very Tense
  Lathyrus—Chick pea (homeopathic)

Deterioration
  Shepard's Purse Tea
>   Two cups a day.

Function
  Vitamin E needed.

Jerks
  Magnesium needed.

Pain
  Vitamin B, E, Calcium Lactate

Spasms, At Night
  Calcium Lactate

Spasms, Daytime
   Magnesium

Twitching
   Scullcap

Weak After Illness
   Almonds
      Eat and add to food and eat.

Weakness
   Shepard's Purse

Muscles, Tendons and Tissues
Injuries
   Comphrey Compresses

Arnica Tincture
      A few drops in water, make compress. Also take a few drops in
      water by mouth.

Daisy Tea
      This is superb. Drink two to three cups a day.

MUSCLE WEAKNESS IN GENERAL
Gentian Tea—½ cup twice a day.

Wormwood with
Lady's Mantle Tea

MUSCLE WEAKNESS IN CHILDREN
Barley Malt

Juniper Berry Branches
      Boil for 45 minutes, strain and then add the tea to bath water. Soak
      for 20 minutes.

MUSCLE WEAKNESS IN SENIOR CITIZEN
Yarrow Tea—2 cups a day.

MYOPIC ASTIGMATISM
Tiger Lily (homeopathic)

N

NARCOTIC POISONING
Bayberry Tea or in capsules.

NAUGHTY CHILDREN
Mallow Leaf Tea
>Add honey to taste.

NAUSEA
Summer Savory—½ teaspoon.

NAUSEA, CONSTANT
Peach Leaf Tea

NECK, ACHES IN
Watch for reproductive organs out of harmony.

NEPHRITIS, ACUTE
Elder Flower Tea—4 cups a day.

NERVES INFECTED AND VERY PAINFUL
Peppermint Tea

Peppermint—locally.

NERVE PAIN IN ARMS AND LEGS
Yarrow Tea in Bath
>One handful Yarrow brewed, strained and added to bath.

NERVE SEDATIVE
Myrtle Tea

NERVE TONIC
Oat Water
>   Add to fruit juice.

>   Barley Water
>   Add to fruit juice.

NERVOUS COMPLAINTS
Motherwort Tea—2 cups a day.

Valerian Root—½ cup twice a day.

NERVOUS EXHAUSTION
Silicon Herbs (see back of book).

NERVOUS HEART
Rue Tea (Not During Pregnancy).

NERVOUS TENSION
Catnip

Mint
>   Make tea and drink one cup as needed.

NERVOUS WEAKNESS AFTER ILLNESS
Scullcap Tea
>   ½ cup three times a day.

NERVOUS AND UPSET
Bugleweed Tea as needed.

NEURALGIA
St. John's Wort in homoepathic form Hypericum.

St. John's Wort
Primula

Passion Flowers—2 cups a day.

Mullein Oil
Yarrow Oil
Chamomile Oil

Thyme Oil
>Mix the oils and apply to pain.

Chamomile Tea

NEURALGIA OF LOWER JAW
Prickly Ash Tea—1 cup a day.

NEURALGIC PAIN
Red Onion
>Make a poultice and apply.

NEURALIGIC PAIN IN ANKLE
Mullein Tea

NEURALGIC PAIN IN RIGHT ANKLE
Yarrow Tea
>Drink and compress.

NEURASTHESIA
Gentian Tea—½ cup twice a day.

Alfalfa Tea—or as tablets.

NERVES
St. John's Wort Oil
>On painful spots.

Green Leaves of Lily Plant
>Tie on painful spots.

NERVES, INFLAMED (Very painful)
Peppermint Tea

Peppermint Lotion

NERVES IN KNOTS
Lily Oil

NERVES, INVOLUNTARY NERVOUS SYSTEM
Ginseng

⅔ of all Nerve Diseases have kidney trouble

Horsetail Tea

NERVOUSNESS
Hops

St. John's Wort

Rosemary
Mix, make tea and drink two cups a day.

NIBBLING HABIT
Alfalfa Tablets

NIBBLING HABIT, TO BREAK HABIT
Bearberry Tea
½ cup three times a day.

NIGHT BLINDNESS
Club Moss Tea—1 cup.

NIGHT SWEATS, PROFUSE
Dandelion Leaf Tea—3 cups.

NOISE, CANNOT BEAR
Nux Vomica (homeopathic)

NOSE, HAS CRUST FORMATION
Buckwheat Grots

NOSEBLEED
Shepards Purse—2 cups a day.

NOSE, BLOWING FREQUENTLY
Couch Grass Tea
Two tablespoons to a cup of water. Drink several cups a day.

NOSE, DRY AND OBSTRUCTED
Elder Flower Tea—2 cups a day.

NOSE (Chronic Nasal Inflamation)
Blood Root Tea—½ cup twice a day.

NUMBNESS OF FINGERTIPS
Lathyrus—Chick Pea (homeopathic)

NUMBNESS OF TONGUE
Lathyrus—Chick Pea (homeopathic)

NURSING, PAIN (Goes from nipple to all over body)
Poke Root Tea/2 cups a day.

O

OBESITY
Raspberry Tea—1 cup

Kelp—2 tablespoons

Fennel Seed Tea—½ cup or more before meals to decrease appetite.
       Do all the above three times a day.

Another recipe
Chickweek Tea—4 cups a day.

Kelp

OBJECTS LOOK DISTORTED IN SIZE
Nutmeg
       ½ teaspoon ground nutmeg in one cup of hot water, sip slowly.

ODOR, CANNOT BEAR
Nux Vomica (homeopathic)

OLD AGE
Sage

Drink one cup of Sage Tea after each meal. I found the following recipe is tasty and invigorating: After work I take one slice of whole grain bread, butter it and sprinkle generously with sage. After eating this all feeling of weariness is gone.

OLD SORES
Plantain Juice

Fresh—applied to the sore and drink Plantain Juice.

OPEN SORES
Lavender Tea Compresses

OSTEOARTHRITIS
Can be helped by feeding the pituitary gland.

OTITIS
Pulsatilla (homeopathic)

OVARIAN CYST
Calendula—2 parts
Yarrow—1 part
Nettle—1 part

Mix and make tea using two tablespoons to one quart of water. Drink one quart a day for four weeks.

OVARIES, SWOLLEN
Potassium
Trace minerals from firewood.

OVERWEIGHT
Celery Seed

Celery, fresh

Lady's Mantle

Cleavers—2 cups a day

Fennel Seed—Takes appetite away

Kelp—Stimulates Glands

Raspberry Leaf Tea

P

PAIN
Yam
> For any kind of pain.

PAIN IN:
Achilles Tendon
> St. Ignatius Bean (homeopathic)

Ankles
> St. John's Wort (homeopathic)

Ankles and Feet
> Poke Root Tea
>> Drink two cups a day and soak feet in Poke Root Tea.

Ankle Joints
> Tiger Lily (homeopathic)

Bones
> Comfrey Root Tea
> Comfrey Root Tincture applied to the painful area.

Breathing
> Iron

Burning
> Vitamin B-12
> Folic Acid

Cramp-like in feet and soles
> Mullein Leaf Tea
> Cabbage compresses

Deep in Head
    Buckwheat as a food.

Facial Muscle
    Vitamin B-12
    Folic Acid

Fingers, Acute
    St. John's Wort

From Hip to Feet
    Cayenne Pepper - in socks

Head (radiating from one point)
    Black Tea—1 cup

Head (with nausea)
    Iris-Blue Flag (homeopathic)

Head
    Lady's Slipper Tea
    (Also called Nerve Root)

    Lavender Tea

    Lavender Oil
        To temples NOT TO BE TAKEN INTERNALLY

    Lavender
        Applied hot will relieve almost any local pain.

    Guarana Tea
        One cup when headache starts.

Pain in Head points to the following trouble:

Back of head
    Liver and gallbladder

Front of Head
    Kidney, bladder

Middle
    Intestinal Trouble

On One Side or The Other Side
    Allergic Reaction to Something

Right Sided
  Celadine Tea—1 cup a day.

Heat in Soles
  Mugwort

Heel
  Club Moss Tea—1 cup a day.

Heels when sitting
  ' Valerian Tea—one cup a day.

Joint
  Comfrey Root Tea
      Apply and drink.

Comfrey Root Tincture—Apply.

Joints
  Avocado Seeds—chop 4 seeds
  Horsetail Grass—three ounces
      Boil together in one quart water, down to one pint. Add rubbing
      alcohol and use as a linament.

Lavender
      In bags, applied hot will quickly relieve almost any localized pain.

Baking Soda
  Rub on painful muscles.

Joints, Ankle
  Tiger Lily (homeopathic)

Left Side of Head
  Alfalfa Tablets

Liver, Right Side of
  Yucca Tablets

Neck
  Comfrey Root Tea

  Rose Petals

  Red Clover Tops

  Orange Blossoms, Nutmeg, Mace

Pectoral Muscle
   Echinacea Tea—or in capsules

Rheumatic, Cramplike
   Horsetail Tea—or in capsules.

Right Side of Liver Area
   Yucca Tablets

Shifting
   Poke Root Tea
   Yam

Spine without any other reason
   Pink Root as a tea ½ cup twice daily.

Shoulder, Right with Stiffness to Raise Arm
   Poke Root Tea—2 cups a day.

Shoulder—Arm Syndrome
   Iron
   Copper
   Vitamin B-1
   Folic Acid

Stump (Amputated)
   Vitamin B-1
   Vitamin B-12

Toes
   St. John's Wort

Wandering Nature
   Echinecea

PAINFUL PILES
Silicon Herbs (see back of book)

PALSEY
Onion
      Eat one raw onion a day.

PANCREAS
Red Beets

Nutmeg

Use freshly ground and store it only briefly for Nutmeg becomes rancid easily and does not work.

Calamus Root

Chew the root.

PANCREAS FOOD

Leeks

Use them in soups, steamed or boiled in salads. Leeks stimulate insulin production.

Green Beans

Boil Green Beans in plenty of water until done. Drink the beanwater, one cup a day and eat one cup of cooked green beans a day to strengthen the pancreas.

PANCREAS, WEAK

Iris-Blue Flag (homeopathic)

Oat Straw Tea

Has to be boiled. This increases insulin. Drink two to three cups a day.

PARALYSIS

Lavender Oil—NEVER TO BE TAKEN INTERNALLY

Lavender Oil is of service when rubbed on externally; for stimulation of paralyzed limbs. Lavender applied hot will relieve almost any local pain. Lavender Tea is excellent for relieving headaches due to fatigue. Also Lavender Oil rubbed on the temples will help to relieve headaches.

PARALYSIS OF FACIAL MUSCLES

Vitamin B-12
Folic Acid

On Left Side

Prickly Ash Tea—1 cup twice a day.

After Stroke

Tobacco Water

Wash limbs with Tobacco Water.

Of Tongue
  Prickly Ash
    Chew herb

PELVIC PORTAL, CIRCULATION TO
Tansy Tea—½ cup twice a day.

PELVIC PORTAL CONGESTION
Stone Root

Callinsonia

PERSPIRATION
Pleuresy Root
Linden Flowers
    Make tea, sweeten with honey and drink 8 ounces.

PHLEBITIS
Witchhazel

Vitamin E

Vitamin C

Bioflavenoids

Collinsonia

White Oak Bark Tea for Trace Minerals
    One to two quarts tea.

Reduce Salt

Reduce Meat

Black Radish and Parsley
    Two tablets every hour.

Golden Seal Root Capsule
    One every hour.

Cottage Cheese Compresses

PIMPLES
Lemon Verbena Tea
>Dampen a clean cloth and scrub face vigorously. Repeat for nine days and see an improvement.

PITUITARY, DEFICIENT OR WEAK
Wild Cherry Bark Tea
>One cup a day.

Cherry Juice

POISON OAK
White Oak Bark Tea—applied.

POLIO MYELITIS
Lathyrus—Chick Pea (homeopathic)

POLLUTION
Willow Leaf Tea—2 cups a day.

POLYPS IN MOUTH
Horsetail

POLYPS IN NOSE
Oak Bark Tea (strong)
>Sniffle it up into nose several times a day.

POTASSIUM, LACK OF
Lady's Mantle

Banana

PREVENTION FOR COLD
Thyme Tea
>One cup a day feeds the thymus gland.

PREVENTION OF INFECTIOUS DISEASES
Pimpernel or
Juniper Berries
>This was used to prevent plague in the Middle Ages.

PREVENTION OF THE A.I.D.S. Virus

A new virus has come over the earth. This virus is a *lipid* coated virus. There are several lipid coated viruses known as Epstein-Barr, CMV and the A.I.D.S. Virus, H.T.L.V., A.R.C. Please folks, protect yourself from this killer.

Take one tablespoon lecthin granules and one egg yolk (fresh), mix thoroughly and add to juice (No citrus) or water or skim-milk. Do this twice a week. This will liquify the virus and it cannot attach.

PROFUSE FLOW OF SALIVA
Iris-Blue Flag (homeopathic)

PROLAPSED ORGANS
Lady's Mantle Tea
>Drink three to four cups a day. One teaspoon per cup of boiling water.

PROLAPSED UTERUS
Oak Bark Tea—1 cup twice a day.

PROLAPSED WOMB
Squaw Weed

Life Root
>One teaspoon five times a day.

PROSTATE ENLARGED
Cough Grass

Echinacea—2 capsules three times a day.

Milk Compresses
>Make as you would give a diaper to a baby. Warm the milk (Do Not Boil), soak a turkish/terrycloth (cotton) towel in it and apply as a diaper. Cover with hot water bottle and do place a plastic sheet underneath.

LOSS OF POWER, NEUROTIC
Saw Palmetto

PLEURISY

Pleurisy Root Tea—several cups.

Lady's Mantle Tea—2 cups a day.

Thyme

Fennel

> Make tea; this combination relaxes.

P.M.S.

Cramp Bark Tea—1 cup as needed.

POISON IVY

Rhus Toxicodudron (homeopathic)

White Oak Bark Tea—in bath.

Sassafras Tea—in bath.

Tansy Tea Bath

Epsom Salt

> Wet Epsom Salt and apply to painful area.

PROTEIN DIGESTANT

Sage Tea—1 cup twice a day.

Basil

Celery

> Aids to protein digestion, can increase appetite and is good for mucous, therefore it is used in rheumatic pain, gastric trouble, colds, cough and urinary disorders.

PROTEIN LOCKED

Sage Tea—1 cup twice a day.

PSORIASIS

Cheladonium (homeopathic)

Iris-Blue Flag (homeopathic)

Cheladonium Majus (homeopathic)

Nettle Tea

Calendula Tea

Iodine—1 part (not white)
Castor Oil—4 parts
    Mix and apply to skin once a day.

PUTRIFICATION, ARREST IT
Charcoal

Burnt Toast

PYORRHEA
Golden Seal
Myrrh
    Make tea and hold in mouth several times a day.

Calamus Root
    Chew small pieces several times a day.

    Make your own toothpaste: Powdered Calcium, (Bonemeal is Best)
add: Sage
Myrrh
Golden Seal (very little it is bitter).

R

RADIATION
Clorox
    Add six ounces of Clorox brand bleach to your bath and soak for ten to fifteen minutes.

Willow Leaf Tea
    Drink two cups when fallout is coming down and make a Willow Leaf Tea to put in the bath for children and weak adults.

Salt
Baking Soda
    Add one pound of each (salt and soda) to your bath water and soak for fifteen minutes.

RECTUM, ACHING
Spikenard Tea—½ cup twice a day.

RECTUM, PROLAPSED
Spikenard Tea—½ cup twice a day.

RECTUM, ULCERATED
Chlorophyll
    Either in capsules or in liquid form.

REJUVENATION
H-12 (see back of book)

REPRODUCTION ORGANS, FEMALE, TO STRENGTHEN
Yarrow

Calendula

Nettle

REPRODUCTIVE ORGANS, MALE, TO STRENGTHEN
Saw Palmetto (homeopathic)

RESISTANCE TO DISEASE
Thyme Tea—1 cup a day.

RESISTANCE, LOW
Calcium Herbs (see back of book)

RESPIRATORY AILMENT
Celery Seed Tea

RESPIRATORY TROUBLE
Thyme Tea—several cups a day.

RESTLESSNESS
Nettle Tea—1 to 2 cups a day.

RETAINING NATURAL COLOR OF HAIR
Iodine Herbs (see back of book)

RETINA BLEEDING
Vitamin C

Bioflavenoids

Rutin

Vitamin B-1

Raw Potato Compresses over eye.

Paprika (Hungarian) one teaspoon three times a day.

RHEUMATIC DEAFNESS
Mistletoe (homeopathic)

RHEUMATISM IN UPPER RIGHT SIDE OF BODY
Violet Root Tea

RHINITIS, CHRONIC (Nasal Inflamation)
Blood Root Tea—½ cup twice a day.

RIDGED NAILS
Silicon Herbs (see back of book)

RIGHT SIDED HEADACHES
Calandine Tea—1 cup a day.

RINGING IN EAR
Iris-Blue Flag (homeopathic)

RING WORMS
Blood Root
  Externally apply the strong tea. Peel, rub it on area.

S

SADNESS
Basil Tea
Or sprinkle on food.

SADNESS IN THE MORNING
Club Moss Tea—in the morning.

SALIVA, TO INCREASE
Prickly Ash Tea

Sage—chew leaves.

Cloves—chew.

SALIVA, PROFUSE FLOW
Plantain

Iris-Blue Flag (homeopathic)

SCARS
Peppermint Oil
     Rub on scar.

SCIATICA
Pink Root
St. John's Wart
Cayenne Pepper
Black Tea
     Mix and try a cup.

Elderberry Juice
     A specific for sciatica.

Elderberry Tea
     Also good.

SCIATICA, WORSE IN HOT WEATHER
Mugwort

SEA SICKNESS
Pennyroyal
> Carry it with you when traveling.

SHINGLES, AN INFECTION OF THE NERVE ENDINGS
Home Remedy
> Witch Hazel—4 ounces or
> Spirit of Camphor—4 ounces add
> Oil of Peppermint—8 drops
>> Mix, shake and apply to painful area.

Leeks
> Blend some of the leaves in the blender with a little water and apply to the painful area.

SINGING, DIFFICULTY
Sulphur

SINUS
Grape Juice
> Sip six ounces twice a day for six weeks.

SINEW, TENDONS AND JOINTS, INJURIES TO
Comfrey Root Compresses

SKIN
Combine Comfrey with any good face or hand lotion to produce a product that has been found valuable in removing various imperfections on the skin and will in some instances cause wrinkles to disappear.

SKIN AILMENTS
Slippery Elm
> Make a poultice for many skin ailments such as burns, boils, ulcers and other type wounds.

SKIN, BLOOD PURIFIER FOR
Strawberry Leaves

Primula Officinalis

Nettle

Ground Ivy

SKIN, DRY
Cocoa Butter—1 part
Glycerine—1 part
Lanolin—1 part
Rosewater—1 part
Elder Flower Water—1 part
> Mix and apply to skin daily.

SKIN TROUBLE
Pansy Tea—2 cups a day.

SKIN WITH TUMOR-LIKE ERUPTIONS
Sheep Sorrel
> Wash skin with strong tea.

SLEEPLESSNESS
Dill Oil
> Rub on forehead.

Cowslip
> Sweetened with honey.

Poppy Seed
> Sleep on a pillow of poppy seed to bring tranquility to the body and mind and hasten natural slumber.

Foot Bath
> At night take a hot foot bath, so poisons are elimated. Rub soles of feet with a slice of lemon to give sound sleep after foot bath.

Chamomile Tea

Lemon Balm Tea

SLEEP WALKING
Mugwort Tea

SORE THROAT
Sage Tea—gargle.

SORES, OLD
Plantain Juice
 Fresh on sore or drink Plantain Tea. Also apply.

SPASMS IN BOWELS AFTER FOOD
Valerian Root Tea—½ cup

SPASMS IN BLADDER
Uva Ursi Tea—1 cup three times a day.

SPEAKING, DIFFICULTY
Sulphur herbs

SPLEEN
St. John's Wort Tea—and/or compress.

SPLEEN CONGESTION
Verbena Tea—2 cups.

Enlarged
 Daisy Tea
 Dandelion Tea
  Mix. Two cups a day.

Painful
 Dandelion Tea
 Sorrel Tea
  Mix. Two cups a day.

Soothing
 Inner Bark of the Maple Tree—make a tea.

Swollen
  Poke Root
  Make a poultice.

Eat Red Beets.

SPRING CLEANING
Nettle Tea

Dandelion Tea

SPINE, CURVATURE
Chlorine Herbs (see back of book)

H-12 applied to spine.

SPINE TROUBLE
Scullcap—1 cup 2 times daily.

STIFF NECK
Hawthorne
        When head is drawn to the right side with a stiff neck.

Chickweek—2 cups a day.

Motherwort—1 cup a day.

Capsium—a little bit.

Crampbark—1 cup.

Celandine
        When head is drawn to the left side with a stiff neck.

        Basil Tea—or sprinkle on food.
STIFFNESS WITH SHOUTING PAIN
Vitamin B-12

STIMULANT
Capsium

Horseradish

STITCHES IN CHEST
Clover Tea—2 to 3 cups.

STITCHES BETWEEN THE SHOULDER BLADES
Ranunculus—Buttercup—2 cups a day.

STOMACH
Iron Weed

Anacardium (Cashew Nut)

Calamus Root—uncooked

Cleavers

STOMACH, HEAVINESS
Ginger Tea

STOMACH TROUBLE
Slippery Elm Tea

STOMACH, SOUR
Raw Potatoe Slices—eat.

Charcoal Tablets

STOMACH STRENGTHENING
Whey
> One tablespoon whey three times a day to feed the stomach glands
> and they will work better for you.

STOMACH ULCER
Calamus Root Tea
> Cut root and let stand overnight in water. Then warm it, DO NOT
> BOIL. Sip ½ cup before meals.

Marigold Tea

Yarrow Tea

Nettle Tea

Malva Tea

STOMACH UPSET, NERVES
Cinnamon
>Drink Cinnamon Tea or chew on Cinnamon sticks.

STOMACH, WEAK
Gentian—very little.

Powdered Okra (available in caps)

Slippery Elm Tea

STOOL, WITH GREAT FORCE
Ground Ivy Tea—1 cup

STRENGTHEN VEINS
Agrimony Tea or in capsule form.

Stoneroot Tea or in capsule form.

STROKE
Lavender Tea—2 cups.

Angelica Root Tea—1 cup.

Mustard Seed
>Every morning thoroughly chew one teaspoon of mustard seed.

STUMP PAIN (Amputated)
Comfrey Root Tea

STUTTERING
Eyebright Tea
>Hold in mouth several times a day.

STYE (EYE)
Eyebright (homeopathic if possible)

Castor Oil

Burdock Root Tea
>Drink it and apply.

SUMMER HEAT
Motherwort Tea

SWELLING
Lettuce Water

Over swollen parts of the body, ankles, abdomen, liver and whatnot.

SWOLLEN ANKLES
Potato Peelings

Take a handful of unsprayed potato peelings and cover with two cups of water. Simmer for fifteen minutes and strain. Take two tablespoons of this in a glass of water four times a day for fourteen days. After several days legs and ankles should be more normal size.

SWOLLEN GLAND
Marjorum

Plantain

Make an oil with these and apply. Plantain neutralizes poisons.

SWOLLEN KNEES
Raw Cabbage

Cabbage is terrific for poultices over swollen knees or elbows. Grate two cups of cabbage very fine. Wrap in cloth and apply overnight. Do several nights in a row.

SWOLLEN LEGS
Lady's Mantle

SWOLLEN FINGERS
Iodine Herbs (see back of book)

SWOLLEN OVARIES
Potassium

Trace Minerals from Firewood

SWOLLEN TESTICLES
Potassium

Fenugreek for Trace Minerals

Echinacea in capsule form

T

TACHYCARDIA

Hawthorne

Blessed Thistle

Red Roses

> Mix equal parts, make tea and drink two cups a day.

TAPEWORM

Pomegranate Twigs

> Boil and drink three cups a day during the full moon for three days in a row.

TEARS, EXCESS

Basil

> Compresses over eyes.

TEETH, CLENCHED

Poke Root Tea

> One cup three times a day.

TEETH, LOOSE

Hold warm apple cider vinegar in mouth several times a day.

Sage

> Mixed with honey and hold in mouth.

TEETH, REFILLS (small holes)

Bonemeal

TEETH, SENSITIVE TO COLD

Magnesium

TEETH, STRENGTHENER

Bonemeal

TENDONS, TISSUE AND MUSCLES
Alchemilla Vulgaris

TENDON, BONE, MUSCLE INJURIES
Comfrey Compresses

TENSION, NERVOUS
Catnip
Mint
> Make a tea and drink one cup as needed.

TENSION IN UPPER HALF OF FACE
Violet Leaf Tea

THROAT, SORE
Sage Tea
> Gargle.

Arnica Tincture
> Two to three drops in a tablespoon of warm water.

Sea Salt in
Vinegar Water
> Gargle with.

THROAT, TOO MUCH SALIVA
Calcium

THROAT, (whiter under the chin than on the other parts of the neck
Magnesium

Sulfur

THYMUS SECREATION, INSUFFICIENT
Copper Herbs (see back of book)

THUMB, DRAWN INTO THE PALM
Helleborous

THYROID
Enlarged
  Poke Root Compresses—overnight.

Sluggish
  Kelp
  Seaweed

TIC FEVER
Chaparell
      Three tablets three times a day for one month.

TICKLING COUGH
Club Moss Tea

TONGUE, BURNING
Malva
      Boil and hold a teaspoon in mouth.

TONGUE, NUMB
Lathyrus—Chick Pea (homeopathic)

TONGUE, PARALYZED
Ginger—chew.

Lavender—chew.

TONGUE, SORES ON
Raspberry Leaf Tea
      Hold in mouth several times a day.

TONGUE, WHITE COATED
Peppermint Leaves
      Hold in mouth.

TONIC IN GENERAL
Dogwood Tea

TRAUMA IN EYE (hard blow)
Comfrey Root Compresses

TRENCH MOUTH
Raspberry

Oak Bark
> Make a juice and spray it in mouth.

Raspberry Leaf Tea

TRINCHINOSIS
Oil of Wintergreen

TUMORS
Eggplant peelings boil and take 2 tablespoons 2x daily.

TUMORS, FATTY
Asparagus
> Canned, the cheap ones are best. Blend it and take two tablespoons in the morning and at night. Put it on bread or eat it alone.

TUMORS, FIBROID
Golden Rod

Calendula
Yarrow
Nettle
> Mix and one quart a day for four weeks.

TWITCHING EYELID
Elder Flower Tea
Vitamin B-6

TYMPANITES (Wind)
Dandelion Root or Leaf Tea—after meals.

U

ULCERS
Calendula Tea

Calamus Root—Chew.

ULCERS, DUODENAL
Calendula Root Tea
>Soak root in water overnight. In the morning warm do not boil. Drink ½ cup four or five times a day.

ULCERS, MOUTH
Sage or
Willow Leaves

Blackberry Leaf Tea—hold in mouth.

ULCER, STOMACH
Calamus Root Tea
>Cut and soak the root in water overnight, warm in the morning, do not boil. Drink or rather sip ½ cup before each meal.

ULCERATED WOUNDS
Milk Compresses
>Draw out bacteria so that wounds can heal.

UNDER DEVELOPED MAMMARY GLANDS
Saw Palmetto (homeopathic)

UREA, EXCESSIVE
Senna Leaf Tea

Juniper Berry Tea

See Physician about Magnesium Deficiency.

Horsetail Grass Tea

URINE BURING
Marshmellow Root Tea
>Three or more cups as needed.

URINE, DIABETIC
Dwarf Bean

Uva Ursi Tea—1 cup a day.

Flax Seed Tea—3 cups a day.

URINATION, FREQUENT
Cherry Juice
>One glass three or four times a day.

URINATION, PAINFUL
Marshmellow Root Tea
>Three cups or more as needed.

URTICARIA
Nettle
>One cup three times a day.

URTICARIA, WITH ITCHING AND BURNING
Nettle
Linden Flower
>Make and drink one cup of tea three times a day.

URTICARIA, WITHOUT ITCHING
Nettle

Buttercup
>Make Tea and drink one cup three times a day.

UTERUS
Fig Leaves
>For female trouble, strengthens the lining of the uterus.

UTERUS, BLEEDING
Vitamin B-6 when no other pathological disturbances can be found.

UTERUS, CIRCULATION
Tansy Tea
> ½ cup two times a day.

UTERUS, CRAMPS
Cramp Bark Tea
> ½ cup two times a day.

UTERUS, ENLARGED
Yarrow Tea

UTERUS, HEMORRHAGE
Ice
> To the nipples will stop uterus bleeding at once.

UTERUS, PROLASPED
Oak Bark

Squaw Root

Life Root
> Combine and make strong tea. One teaspoon five times a day.

UTERUS, SORE
Linden Flower Tea with honey

VACCINATION, ILL EFFECTS
Thuja (homeopathic)

VARICOSE VEINS
Marigold
> One ounce powdered flowers and stems with one plant of boiling water, allow to cool and apply directly to various affected parts of the body such as varicose veins, chronic ulcers and similar ailments.

Oak Bark Tea Compress—overnight.

Plantain
Yarrow
Mullein
Calendula
    Mix, make tea and drink three cups a day.

Calendula Salve—apply.

Cottage Cheese Compress
    If possible all night or just for several hours. Do this every night
    until gone.

VARICOSE VEINS IN PREGNANCY
Daisy Tea

VARICOSE VEINS IF PURPLE
Horse Chestnut

VEIN, STRENGTHENER
Agrimony Tea or in capsule form.

Stoneroot Tea or in capsule form.

VENOUS ENGORGMENT
Stone Root

Callinsonia
    Two caps twice a day.

VERMIFUGE
Wormgrass
    Also called American Wormwood. Take two to three cups around
    the full moon.

VERTIGO
Crab Apples
    Boil and eat a teaspoon every hour.

VIOLENCE
Larkspur Tea
> One tablespoon five times a day.

VIOLENT DISPOSITION
Livah* Tradename

Golden Rod

Golden Seal

Cloves

VIRUS INFECTION
Calendula Tea

VOICE, HOARSE
Mullein Leaf Tea—as needed.

VOID, MUST DO HURRIEDLY
Chick Pea (homeopathic)

Cherry Juice—2 cups a day.

W

WALKING, CANNOT ON UNEVEN GROUND
Tiger Lily (homeopathic)

WARTS
Fenugreek Seed
> Soak seed in water until it makes a mucilage-like ointment. Apply
> to the wart and let dry. Use once a day until the wart disappears.

Dandelion Juice
> Apply topically.

Milkweed Juice
 Same.

Thuja (homeopathic)

Willow Leaf (fresh)
 Squeeze the juice on the wart.

WARTS, PLANTAR
Chalk
 Oil a piece of cloth and grate regular blackboard chalk over the oiled area and apply it over night. Do this for fourteen days.

WATER RETENTION IN STOMACH AND INTESTINES
Woodruff Tea—3 cups a day.

Nettle—2 parts
Uva Ursi—1 part
 Mix, make tea and drink four cups a day to eliminate excess water from the cells.

WEAK BONES
Fenugreek Seed
 In tablet or capsule form.

WEAKNESS
Ginseng Root

WEAKNESS IN SENIOR CITIZEN
Yarrow Tea
 Two cups a day.

WEIGHT LOSS (to Reduce)
Angelica—2 parts
Caraway—1 part

WILLPOWER
Calcium

WORMS
Pumpkin Seeds

> Eat ½ cup pumpkin seeds a day, especially before a meal on an empty stomach. Worms are stripped from their protective skin by eating pumpkin seed.

Birch Leaves or Bark

Blue Cohosh

Quassia Root Tea—weak to drink.

Quassia Foot Bath

Calcium

> When worms are repeated.

WORMS, TAPEWORM
Pomegranate Twigs

> Boil and drink three cups a day during the full moon for three days in a row.

WORRY IN AGED
Larkspur Tea

> One teaspoon to a cup of boiling water. Drink one cup four times a day.

WRINKLES
Cowslip Oil

WRINKLES, FOREHEAD
Helleborous

WRINKLES, HANDS AND FEET
Violet Root

White Helleborus Tea—wash in.

Chapter II

How to Make Your Own
Healing Oils

Take 2 handfuls of fresh herbs or
1 handful of dried herbs
Cover with olive oil.
Let it stand in a warm place for 14 days.
Stir it once in awhile and after fourteen days simmer oil with the herbs for 15 minutes, strain. Squeeze the last drop of oil out of the mixture. Again fill with one handful of dried herbs in the leftover oil and placing it on a warm place repeat the procedure. After 14 days, bring it to a boil and simmer it again for 15 minutes. Strain and squeeze out the last drop of oil. There is not much left, however the oil is mighty potent and you only need a few drops. (I use a double boiler.)

Calendula Oil is good for boils and everything that does not want to heal.

Dill Oil can be rubbed on all aching parts. Moisten the forehead to induce sleep. Very beneficial for bladder and kidney discomfort as also: tonsils, liver, spleen and/or injuries, when Dill Oil is applied to the skin it will release the tenderness a great deal.

Juniper Oil is very good for cramps in legs and pain in hips, also for paralysis. Mash Juniper Berries and proceed with the Healing Oil recipe. Rub into painful area.

Lily Oil made from fresh Lily Flowers, helps spasms, tendons, wrinkles and scars.

Peppermint Oil is helpful for frozen fingers or ears. Rub on scars or callouses.

Chamomille Oil for cramplike pains. Rub baby's tummy with it, take a few drops for indigestion.

HOW TO MAKE TINCTURES

Take any herb, preferably fresh and place in a jar that has a tight fitting lid. Cover with 80 proof alcohol (not rubbing alcohol) and let it sit in a warm place for 10 to 14 days, stirring once in a while. After 14 days strain and fill into bottles. Use only small amounts, for it is potent.

Chapter III

Categorizing Herbs

We are accustomed to categorizing our lives and also our environments. Reluctantly I do so with herbs—the medicine of the ages, the medicine of God's drugstore.

This outline I am giving here is only a small portion of herbs in your vicinity. By walking through the meadows you will find the iron herbs, the magnesium herbs, and so on, easily.

All herbs have iron but some have more than others and give off the vibration of iron more readily than others do.

Working with herbs we work with vibrations. Herbs are in tune with the universe and in tune with Mother Earth.

Willingly, the plants will give up this vibration to heal us. The most powerful herbs for healing are the herbs which grow in your vicinity. Malva leaves from your backyard are more powerful to your ailing colon than the most expensive herbals from India and the dandelion in your frontyard is more beneficial to you than the Chinese herbs which are so healing to the Chinese.

The trouble is that we have not studied our own herbs well enough and we have to rely on someone else's knowledge of herbology.

Out of my personal experience I relate this example to you. The chaparrel bush is a unique bush of the desert. Remaining always shiny green in the hear, this bush does not seem to be bothered by the waterless condition of the desert. It is the "heal all" of the American Indians.

Easily it can be compared with the most beautiful herbs from the Alps in healing quality.

Chaparell is a cleanser, a detoxifier, a healer. It takes fever away and does all of this in a short time—fast and efficiently.

When a person who has just come from China or Switzerland drinks a cup of chaparell tea it acts like poison to them. The vibration of chaparell is so foreign to them they have first to get accustomed to American soil, sun, and food before it is beneficial in healing their fever.

Calcium Herbs are:

Chamomile	Dandelion
Caraway Seeds	Dill
Chives	Horsetail
Cleavers	Pimpernel
Coltsfoot	Tormentil Root

CALCIUM HERBS: May help in bone and teeth conditions, impoverished blood, asthma, overweight, increases resistance, can strengthen all body functions and nervous conditions, increase endurance and vitality.

Chlorine Herbs are:

Fennel	Plantain
Golden Seal	Uva Ursi
Myrrh	Watercress
Nettles	Wintergreen

CHLORINE HERBS: May be helpful in sinus trouble, Bright's disease, magnetism, pyorrhea, bloated abdomen, purifying the blood, cleansing the arteries, cleaning the lymphatic system.

Copper Herbs are:

Dandelion	Salep
Devil's Bit	Sheep Sorrel
Liverwort	

COPPER HERBS: May help to overcome chronic gastric indigestion, gall bladder troubles, insufficient bile secretion, insufficient thymus secretion, low blood sugar, spleen troubles, water retention in tissue.

Fluorine Herbs are:

Corn Silk	Plantain
Dill	Thyme
Horsetail	Watercress
Oats	

FLUORINE HERBS: May be helpful in weakened eyesight, old age problems, skin disorders, broken bones (repair), curvature of spine. Helps prevent pyorrhea, gives resistance to disease.

Iodine Herbs are:

Algae
Dulse
Iceland Moss
Irish Moss
Kelp

Mustard
Nettles
Parsley
Seawrack

IODINE HERBS: May be helpful in goiter, retaining natural color in hair, obesity, proper development in teenagers, healthy nerves, protects body from body toxins, protects brain from body toxins.

Iron Herbs are:

Burdock
Dandelion
Huckleberry Leaves
Irish Moss
Meadow Sweet

Sheep Sorrel
Silver Weed
Stinging Nettle
Strawberry Leaves
Yellow Dock

IRON HERBS: May help in anemia, weakness in old age, shortness of breath, fever of all kinds, give resistance to all kinds of contagious diseases, increase physical power, increase mental power, and strengthen the liver.

Magnesium Herbs are:

Bone Comfort
Broom Tops
Carrot Leaves
Devil's Bit
Meadowsweet

Mullein Leaves
Nettles
Primrose
Walnut Leaves

MAGNESIUM HERBS: May help in tooth decay, irritability, poor circulation, tired blood, nervous prostration, backward children, dull adults, and remove toxins from our bodies. Help in excess acidity and insomnia.

Manganese Herbs are:

Burdock	Strawberry Leaves
Kelp	Wintergreen
Sheep Sorrel	Yellow Dock

MANGANESE HERBS: May help in neuritis, mental instability, sorrow, emotional shock, will aid in reducing, give mental alertness, improve sterility, and poor joints.

Nickel Herbs are:

Algae	Kelp
Bladderwrack	Liverwort

NICKEL HERBS: May help in disorders of the pancreas, weak lining of the intestines, and help the assimilation of nutrients.

Potassium Herbs are:

American Centaury	Plantain Leaves
Carrot Leaves	Primrose Flowers
Comfrey	Summer Savory
Couch Grass	Walnut Leaves
Mullein	Yarrow
Oak Bark	

POTASSIUM HERBS: May help in diseases of the lung and chest, liver disorders, spleen disorders, constipation, brain and nerves, acid stomach, heart muscles, skin eruptions, failure of sores to heal.

Phosphorous Herbs are:

Calamus	Marigold Flowers
Chickweed	Rhubarb
Dill	Sorrel
Licorice Root	Watercress

PHOSPHOROUS HERBS: May be helpful in development of the sixth sense, body poise, electro-magnetic efficiency, nervous disorders in heart and stomach, neuritis, nourish brain, prevent fatigue. All indoor workers need them.

Silicon Herbs are:

Chickweed
Corn Silk
Flax Seed
Horsetail

Lamb's Quarter
Oat Straw
Red Raspberry Leaves
Sunflower Seeds

SILICON HERBS: May be helpful in preventing infections, retarding cancerous growth, soft bones, nervous exhaustion, soft teeth, ridged nails, bad complexion.

Sodium Herbs are:

Apple Tree Bark
Celery Seed
Cleavers
Dill
Fennel Seed

Huckleberry Leaves
Meadow Sweet
Mistletoe
Stinging Nettle

SODIUM HERBS: May help in hardening of the arteries, diabetes, gallstones, arthritis, bladder stones, old age retarding, old age deposits.

Sulphur Herbs are:

Coltsfoot
Eyebright
Fennel
Meadow Sweet
Mullein
Pimpernel

Plantain Leaves
Scouring Rush
Shepherd's Purse
Stinging Nettle
Watercress

SULPHUR HERBS: May be helpful in dissolving the acids in the system, an antiseptic for the alimentary canal, warming the body and the feet, giving energy and high spirits, and strengthening the tissues, for impure blood, leukemia, hemmorhoids, septecemia.

Zinc Herbs are:

Horsetail   Shepherd's Purse
Paprika

ZINC HERBS: May be helpful in a weak pancreas in diabetics, failing eyesight due to insulin, flatulency due to weak pancreas, prostate troubles and ill natured tumors.

Master Formula
H_{12}
for
Old Age and Other
Symptoms

Old age can start as early as age twenty-two and as late as age seventy. Old age is not determined by chronological age, but is determined by the slowing down of glandular functions. It is a filling up of the arterial system with slush and deposits, a breakdown of bodily functions singularly or all together. It is a let down of mental activity and mental capacity. Old age is an attitude, "I don't want to start anything new." Old age begins with lassitude, onesidedness, with failure to recognize the challenge which life has to offer. Old age is a letdown of self-discipline and a letdown of enthusiasm. These are attributes of "Old Age," and you find them in all age groups. Master Formula H_{12} will change this quickly.

The Master Formula H_{12} is an energy-giving formula, which increases the strength of the mind, improves the memory, eliminates depression and anxiety. H_{12} increases the ability to function physically. The Formula acts at the inter-cellular level and restores cells to normal and youthful functions. It also acts on the electro-magnetic ion function of the cells.

Master Formula H_{12} provides a balance between the many stresses of life in today's society. The herbs also bring about the balance in the nervous system, thus releasing energies for physical activity. H_{12} is an anti-aging formula, restoring grey hair and relieving scores of old age aches and pains, depressions and fatigue. It is a most valuable formula to keep arteries clean and youthful and the mind sharp.

This Master Formula H_{12} is handed down through the centuries. It should be used by any age group, particularly now while fallout and environmental toxins destroy our resistance to diseases.

Soon you will find that
    *Aches and pains will be gone
    *Sorrow will go from your doorstep
    *Paralysis will have no place in your body
    *Arteries will be clean and elastic
    *Stomachaches will be a thing of the past
    *Gallbladder and liver resume their responsibility
    *Hearing will be improved
    *Eyesight will be improved
    *Your memory will return
    *Happiness will enter your home

These are the ingredients for Master Formula H_{12}
    Angelica Root
    Apple Tree Bark and Root
    Burdock Root
    Cascara Sagrada
    Calamus Root
    Gentian
    Myrrh
    Peachbark
    Pimpernell
    Rhubarb Root
    Senna Leaves
    Tormentill Root

Recipe

Take 2 ounces of H_{12} and pour 1 qt 80 proof alcohol over it. Let it sit on the window sill for 10 days. Shake every day once or twice. After 10 days strain the fluid off and fill in small bottles. Pour another pt. of 80 proof over the herbs and let sit for 3 days. Then strain and squeeze the herbs as dry as you can preserving every drop of goodness. This second harvest you use for external purposes. It is darker and thicker than the first part. Keep in closed containers.

The ready-made herb mixture is scientifically balanced and available at your health food store or order from New Age Foods, 1122 Pearl St., Boulder, Colo. 80302.

Dosage

(1) For old age symptoms
    1 teasp. in some water 3 times daily.
(2) To keep environmental poisons out
    1 tsp. in water twice daily.
(3) In acute illness with cold symptoms
    1 Tbsp. in water or juice 3 times daily.
(4) Emotional upset
    2 tsp. in warm water.
(5) Ill natured tumors, make compresses over them.
(6) Bellyache in children
    moisten a cottonball with the solution and with a
    bandaid tie over belly button
(7) Put it over the spine, the limbs,
    wherever needed by drops only.
(8) Rub it on the forehead for clearer eyes.
(9) Tie a cottonball with the solution
    on nape of neck for better brain functioning
(10) Drop it into your ear for your hearing, 1 drop only.
(11) On the soles of your feet it will reach all the nerves in
    your body

(12) Rub on chest when coughing
(13) Moisten cloth with H-12 and lay over eyelids when eyes are inflamed.
(14) Many of us suffer from fluid retention. Try one teaspoon H-12, three times daily in water or juice.
(15) Apply to hemorroids with a cottonball.
(16) Depression and melancholy are lessened by taking one teaspoon H-12 twice a day or more often.
(17) Put H-12 on corns and cover with a bandaid.
(18) One teaspoon H-12 in a little water helps digestion and decreases gas formation.

Arteriosclerosis

This term is applied to a pathological condition in which there is thickening, hardening and loss of elasticity of the walls of blood vessels, especially the arteries; in short, it is hardening of arteries.

If hardening of arteries takes place around the heart, open-heart surgery is given. In case hardening of arteries is all over in legs, arms, heart and brain (loss of memory, stroke), chelation therapy may be suggested. In both procedures we have to face side effects.

God in His grace gave us herbs to clear the plague and deposits out of the arteries. To return arteries to a youthful state, to make them elastic and new, try Our Lord's Formula:

Before each meal, 3 times daily, take

1 caps. Equisitum with Silica

2 caps. hawthorn berries

(Now available in one formula called Circu-Flow.)

2 tblsp. aloe vera gel or juice in water or apple juice.

Do this for one month and then have your physician recheck the health of your arteries. If it is not all gone, repeat. Do not eat heavy meals and no potato chips, heavy cakes, alcohol or strong coffee.

Yoghurt and applesauce is a specific to clear arteries and also to keep them clean after the four weeks are over.

The product Equisitum is made in France. It is horsetail made in a specific way. Just to drink a cup of horsetail tea or take horsetail herb will *not* have the desired effect, and you lose time and money.

Heart tonic

The following recipe comes from the great mystic of the Middle Ages Hildegard von Bingen.

Her knowledge of herbs was hidden for many years. It is the work of Dr. G. Hertzka that this writing comes to light.

Take 10 longstemmed parsley cut into ½ inch pieces (leaves and stems are used) and cover the 1 qt natural white wine. Add 1 tablespoon apple cider vinegar and bring this to boil. Simmer for 10 minutes and then add ¾ cup good honey. Now boil again for another 5 min. Strain the wine and fill hot into sterile bottles. Close bottles tightly or set in refrigerator. (caution: wine will run over easily while heating, so stay with it).

Whenever you feel weakness, or aches around heart, or you are overworked take 3 tablespoons from this tonic 2-3 times daily. Parsley wine strengthens heart-nerves, heartmuscle and your heart's entire function becomes stabilized.

Balancing Herb Formulas

I used to mix herbs without rhyme or reason. "If mullein is good for the lungs," I said, "then why not add something else like shave grass for the kidney and peppermint for taste?" Then I met Rev. Dr. Houston who taught me how to mix herbs properly.

"Herbs have a delicate vibration," he said. "By blending herbs together which do not enhance the harmony with each other and for each other, you end up with a dead formula." He also said, "You end up with a dead formula when you take just a teaspoon too much of one item or another. You end up with a dead formula if you do not mix them well afterwards."

The healing of herbs is a blending of vibrations with each other and with the one to be healed; the product has to be well-balanced in order to accomplish this. Chemicals do not have to be well-balanced because chemicals have another purpose and heal on another level.

It is just as it is with people. A well-balanced person can be an immense blessing to their environment. Why is this so? Is it because of the minerals calcium or magnesium or any other minerals or vitamins? No, it is because of the person's life force energy. They manage to balance in themselves the *life energy which makes them balanced.* So it is with herb formulas. They have to be balanced carefully to be a blessing to mankind. Mr. Kroeger invented a device to measure the herb energies. In this way herb formulas can be balanced to the finest point possible. The following **balanced herb formulas** are available in every Health Food Store in America. Ask for information at New Age Food, 1112 Pearl Str., Boulder, Colorado 80302.

Hanna's Herb Formulas

BIO-PEP
Gotu Kola, Yarrow, Yerba Santa,
Bee Pollen, PABA (Para Amino Benzoic Acid)
> An excellent, stimulating and subtle combination to balance the aura and give a rejuvenating feeling to the body. Aura food.

BLACK RADISH & PARSLEY
Black Radish, Parsely
> Helpful for low energy from infections, sore throats. Transmutes strep infection.

BLOOD CLEANSER
Yellow Dock, Cramp Bark,
Yarrow, Milkweed, Tansy Flower,
Plantain, Sail Tobacco
> Often used with cleansing diets for purification of the blood stream. Combined with foongoos for extra effect.

BONE COMFORT
Rose Petals, Dittany of Crete,
Red Clover Tops, Orange Blossoms, Nutmeg
> Often used with calcium as a tonic for bones and teeth. Helpful for aching or broken bones and poor absorption of calcium.

CHEM-X
Black tea, Condurango Bark,
Red Clover Tops, Yellow Dock, Paprika,
Chaparral, Spikenard
> Transmutes chemical deposits. Helpful for fatigue from exposure to chemical pollutants, smoke and aromatic hydrocarbons.

D-BETS
Bean Leaves, Blueberry Leaves,
Paprika, Turmeric, Bittersweet Root
> Food for the pancreas. Helpful for chronic blood sugar problems.

ENERGY FOOD
Chia Seed, Kola Nut, Saw Palmetto
>An excellent strengthening stimulant for keen alertness while driving or studying. Surprisingly strong, safe, natural, not habit forming. For mental clarity from exhaustion.

ENZ
Pine, Myrrh, Catnip, Mullein,
Mugwort, Chamomile
>makes your digestive system work as it did in your teenage years. Our all herbal enzyme.

ENVIRONMENTAL CLEANSE
Taurine, Borage, Cleavers
>Transmutes environmental poisons.

FOON-GOOS
Alfalfa Seed, Blessed Thistle,
Golden Seal Root
>A powerful food combination often used with and after antibiotics. Transmutes fungus infection.

FOON-GOOS II
Blessed Thistle, Golden Seal,
Crampbark, Milkweed, Tansy, Bentonite
>For cellulite deposits or fatty tumors on your body. Also Candida.

G'ALL
Red Clover Tops, Damiana,
Golden Seal, Pennyroyal Leaves, Gotu Kola
>Helpful for chronic gall bladder problems. Releases constipation due to lack of bile.

HEARTWARMER
Mistletoe, Broomtops, Hawthorn,
Chickweed, Buchu
>An excellent food for the heart, especially for high stress. Strengthens the circulatory system.

HERBAL CHELATION
Equisetum Concentrate, Hawthorn
Berries, Quaw Bark
> For Arteriosclerosis. A great combination for when arteries fill with plaque.

IN-FLU
Lemon Peel, Chamomile, Thyme,
Capsicum, Coltsfoot, Yerba Santa,
Eucalyptus, Wahoo, Lungwort
> Helpful for fevers, flus, lung and sinus congestion. An excellent help during viral invasions.

INFLAME
Dandelioin, Fennel Seed, Mugwort,
Horehound, Rosemary
> Helpful for joint pain where constant disturbances and friction may result in inflamation.

KANTITA
Condurango, Yellow Dock, Red Clover
> Transmutes Candida Albicans fungus especially after a long run down condition, antibiotics, or not taking care of yourself. Combine with Foongoos II.

KOL-ESTER
Bethroot, Malefern, Calamus,
Okra, Rhubarb
> An excellent addition used to check cholesterol buildup.

LIV-AH
Golden Rod, Golden Seal, Cloves
> Often taken with liver cleansing diets. Strengthens liver and digestive functioning.

MEN'S SPECIAL
Black Walnut Powder, Saw Palmetto, Cornsilk
> An excellent food for prostate strengthening. Most often used by concerned men over 45. Helpful for impotence and weakened energy.

119

METABOLIZER
Yellow Dock, Uva Ursi, Cleavers,
Golden Seal, Blood Root, Oak Bark, Lycopodium
> Helpful in cleansing the glandular system, balancing thyroid and other glands. Helps with weight problems.

METALINE
Pumpkin Seed, Okra, Rhubarb Root,
Cayenne Pepper, Red Cabbage, Dulse
> Used by people concerned about heavy environmental fallout, smoke, and metals contamination. An improvement of a formula of long standing.

THE MOVER
Marshmallow, Rhubarb, Onion,
Pink Root, Wahoo
> A mild, non-addicting, gentle mover to help those with a sluggish eliminative system.

NEPTUNE
Parsley, Parsley Root, Echinacea
> A mild kidney tonic using herbs of reputed diuretic qualities. Helpful in strengthening the water element.

POL-X
Willow Leaves, Milksugar,
Thyme, Cinnamon
> Transmutes pollution, X-rays, and radiation causing toxic build-up.

PRETTY EYE
Witch Hazel, Rue, Angelica, Golden Seal
> Often used with diet and exercise by people feeling pressure and clouded vision. Helpful for strengthening the eyes.

R.Q.
(READ QUICK)
Dulse, Eyebright, Gotu Kola
> Helpful for mental alertness, mental stamina, clear thinking.

RASCAL
Pumpkin Seeds, Garlic,
Cranberry Bush, Capsicum, Thyme
> A strong treat for unwanted visitors in the alimentary canal.
> Wormifuge.

RUMAFIX
Yucca Extract, Black Walnut,
Wormwood, Fenugreek, Yellow Dock.
> Yucca is the primary ingredient of this food. It is reputed to
> be useful in relieving aches and pains in joints and muscles.

SERENITY
Rosemary, Thyme, Black Cohosh,
Burdock Root, Bethroot
> For nerves in collision. Helpful in soothing nerve tissue, for
> insomnia, hysteria.

SOUND BREATH
Garlic, Rose Hips, Rosemary,
Echinacea, Thyme
> Often used by runners and people trying to build up their wind
> and oxygenation capacities. Lung troubles.

STUFFY
Horseradish, Lettuce, Vitamin C,
Peppermint, Wood Betony
> Helpful for chronic sinus congestion.

TOM-EE
Marjoram, Chamomile, Meadowsweet,
Spearmint, Gentian Root
> A delicious blend pleasing to the stomach. Builds digestive
> energy.

UPLIFT

Lecithin, Licorice Root, Anise

>Often used as a long term food to help combat the moodiness and depressions associated with low blood sugar.

VYREN

Lettuce, Basil, Raspberry Leaves

>A trinity of simple but recognized herbs. Most often taken to help ward off infectious indications.

WOMEN'S GOLD

Licorice Root, Yarrow, Comfrey,
Yellow Dock, Dandelion Root

>Used mostly by young women to strengthen the female system. An excellent combination for many female difficulties.

WORMWOOD

Wormwood, Black Walnut, Cloves

>For long slimy invaders in the large intestines. Wormifuge.